# Understanding S

# Understanding Sexuality

## Third Edition

DEREK LLEWELLYN-JONES

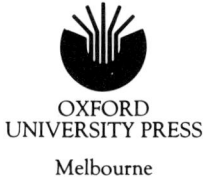

OXFORD
UNIVERSITY PRESS

Melbourne

OXFORD UNIVERSITY PRESS AUSTRALIA

Oxford   New York   Toronto
Delhi   Bombay   Calcutta   Madras   Karachi
Petaling Jaya   Singapore   Hong Kong   Tokyo
Nairobi   Dar es Salaam   Cape Town
Melbourne   Auckland
and associated companies in Berlin   Ibadan

OXFORD is a trademark of Oxford University Press

*First published 1980; reprinted 1981
2nd edition 1984; reprinted with corrections 1985, 1986
3rd edition 1988*

*End of chapter activities
Anne Mulholland
Lawrence St Leger
Seconded from the Education Department to the
Social Biology Resources Centre, Carlton, Victoria*

NATIONAL LIBRARY OF AUSTRALIA CATALOGUING-IN
PUBLICATION DATA

Llewellyn-Jones, Derek, 1923–
Understanding sexuality.

   3rd ed.
   Bibliography.
   Includes index.
   ISBN 0 19 554928 7.

   1. Sex instruction for youth. I. Title.

612'.6

Cover illustration: detail from
sketch for *Children in the Street* (n.d.)
by V. G. O'Connor (1918–   , Australian)
Oil on cardboard, 10.3 × 14.2 cm
Courtesy of Mrs Atida Levine

Designed by Ron Hampton
Illustrations by Juli Kent-Corston
Cartoons by Ben O'Hagen
Typeset by Abb-typesetting Pty Ltd, Collingwood, Victoria
Printed by Globe Press Pty Ltd, Brunswick, Victoria
Published by Oxford University Press,
253 Normanby Road, South Melbourne, Australia

# CONTENTS

# PREFACE

## Learning about human sexuality

When you hear the word 'sex', or 'sexuality', what kind of image is conjured up in your imagination? Many people associate the word with the image of a couple having sexual intercourse. In other words, they associate sexuality only with a physical action.

Sexuality comprises far more than that. It is the sum of a person's inherited make-up, knowledge, experiences, attitudes and behaviour as they relate to being a man or a woman. It includes those ways of behaving which enrich the personality and increase the love between people.

Human sexuality is as much psychological as it is physical. It involves the mind and body, so that the image of the couple making love is only one part of being sexual. It involves how you feel towards another person as much as how you make love to another person. It involves being together, touching and exploring each other's bodies to learn the textures and surfaces, the sight and the smell of another person. It involves the action of learning to respect each other's attitudes to sexuality. It involves communicating with each other. Communication means far more than just talking. It means that you listen to the person, make an effort to understand what the person says, and respond appropriately. Human sexuality means that you find pleasure and enjoyment with another person. You may have arguments and disagreements, but essentially sexuality is pleasurable.

Humans are never non-sexual beings. Babies get pleasure from fondling or rubbing their genitals. Children get pleasure from sexual games.

At puberty a person's sexuality suddenly receives a great boost, as the male and female sex hormones begin to circulate in the bodies of boys and girls. From puberty on, humans are strongly sexual beings. A person's sexuality ends only with that person's death.

Until recently human sexuality was not thought a suitable subject for investigation or discussion. Medical scientists who tried to investigate human sexuality were treated with suspicion. Today, however, the importance of understanding human sexuality is appreciated. Most experts agree that learning about sexuality should start long before a child reaches puberty, so that a foundation for sexual health can be established.

To be sexually healthy you have to learn about and understand human sexuality. You need to know how males and females develop differently in their mother's uterus. You need to understand the differences in behaviour of boys and girls and how these differences arise. It is possible that substances made by the fetus in the uterus may influence a child's behaviour, as male or female, after birth, but a much stronger influence is the way the baby is treated by its parents as a boy or a girl. You need to understand how teenagers and adults respond to sexual arousal, and the many varieties of that response. You need to know something about pregnancy and family planning and sexually transmitted diseases. You need to be able to understand people whose sexual behaviour is different from yours.

Knowledge and understanding of these matters makes for sexual health.

Who should teach teenagers about sexuality? There has been considerable discussion amongst adults on this matter. Some people believe it should be the parents, some believe that clergymen should be involved. Other people believe that teachers or doctors should teach young people about sexuality.

These discussions are rather pointless because young people learn about human sexuality all the time. They learn about it (often inaccurately) from their friends, they learn about it from television, from the cinema, and from magazines. Unfortunately, what they learn is often distorted and sometimes neither correct not truthful. Learning about sexuality, so that the muddle is cleared and the real facts are shown, should be a partnership between parents, teachers and the student. Many parents are embarrassed to talk to their children about sex, and either say nothing or would prefer teachers to take on the responsibility. Even so, parents, by showing love and understanding, play a crucial part in enabling young people to understand and appreciate their own sexuality and that of others.

Learning about sexuality is being able to talk about sexuality, so that fears and anxieties are removed and tensions are lessened. Many people find that it is difficult to talk about sexuality and that misunderstanding may arise between parents and children or between teachers and students.

One purpose of any educational programme is to reduce misunderstanding and to help people to learn.

It is important to young people to learn about human sexuality, just as they learn about other things. Research, in Great Britain and in the USA, has shown that many of the anxieties, the difficulties and the problems which damage relationships between people arise because of the lack, not the excess, of accurate knowledge about their sexuality.

Healthy sexuality is the integration and expression of the physical, the emotional, the intellectual, the spiritual and the social aspects of a person in ways which enhance the personality and enrich the love between two people.

Derek Llewellyn-Jones
Sydney, 1988

# A note to group leaders

At the end of each chapter there are a number of statements to support and extend the material in the text. These are grouped under three headings, viz. Investigations, Discussions and Activities.

They direct themselves to some of the issues raised in the chapter and encourage students to increase their knowledge and understanding of sexuality by further reading and contact with groups and individuals in the field.

The statements are quite broad, and it is anticipated that they will promote many different lines of research. It is important to realize, however, that the leader or teacher needs to provide guidance beyond that which is contained in the statements. This may occur in the form of devising a strategy, adapting the statement, checking learner understanding of the purpose, etc.

Also, a number of these statements may be inappropriate for some learners, depending on the social context. Leaders are encouraged to respect the learning needs of the student and to be sensitive to the environment in which they work.

The statements will promote peer group discussion and further develop the themes of the text. They are strongly recommended. They were prepared by Anne Mulholland and Lawrence St Leger while working in the Department of Education, Victoria, on secondment to the Social Biology Resources Centre, Carlton, Victoria.

# 1
# CHILDHOOD SEXUALITY

A baby has just been born. It lies between its mother's legs as she lies back, supported by pillows. Its eyes open to a new world. The doctor gives the baby to its mother. She looks between its legs and discovers whether this child she has just given birth to is a girl or a boy.

The only way anyone can tell a baby's sex is by looking at its external sex organs, that is, by looking at its genitals. If you see a penis, you know the baby is a boy. If there is no penis, you know the baby is a girl.

Once the parents know the sex of their baby they begin to treat the boy and girl babies in a slightly different way. From birth the baby begins to learn that he is a boy or that she is a girl.

## Why you were born a boy or a girl

Your body is composed of millions of cells of various kinds, for instance, nerve cells and the cells which make up your skin. Each cell has a central nucleus, and this nucleus contains forty-six rod-like **chromosomes**. The chromosomes carry the characteristics which make you different from everybody else, but more like your parents than strangers. This is because you inherit twenty-three of the chromosomes from your mother and twenty-three from your father.

The forty-six chromosomes are of two kinds. Forty-four of them determine your personal characteristics, such as the colour of your eyes, the shape of your nose, your height and physique. Two chromosomes determine your sex or gender, that is whether you are male or female. If you are female every cell in your body will have forty-four general and two X chromosomes; if you are male every cell will have forty-four general, one X and one Y chromosome.

It is not quite correct to write that all the cells of your body contain forty-six chromosomes. The **sperms**, which are made constantly, after puberty, in a man's **testicles**, contain only twenty-three chromosomes; and the **egg-cells** (called **ova**) found in a woman's **ovaries** contain only twenty-three chromosomes. The reason for this is that when a sperm fertilizes an **ovum**, and a new life starts, the combined chromosomes of sperm and ovum make up the required number characteristic of the human race, namely forty-six.

Each egg-cell contains twenty-two general chromosomes and one sex chromosome, called X, because that is what it looks like.

The sperms also contain twenty-two general chromosomes, and one sex chromosome. Half the sperms contain an X chromosome, and the other half a Y chromosome. Each time a man ejaculates, whether it is during a 'wet dream', by masturbating, or during sexual intercourse, several million **spermatozoa** spurt out of his penis. About half of the spermatozoa have nuclei which contain twenty-two gen-

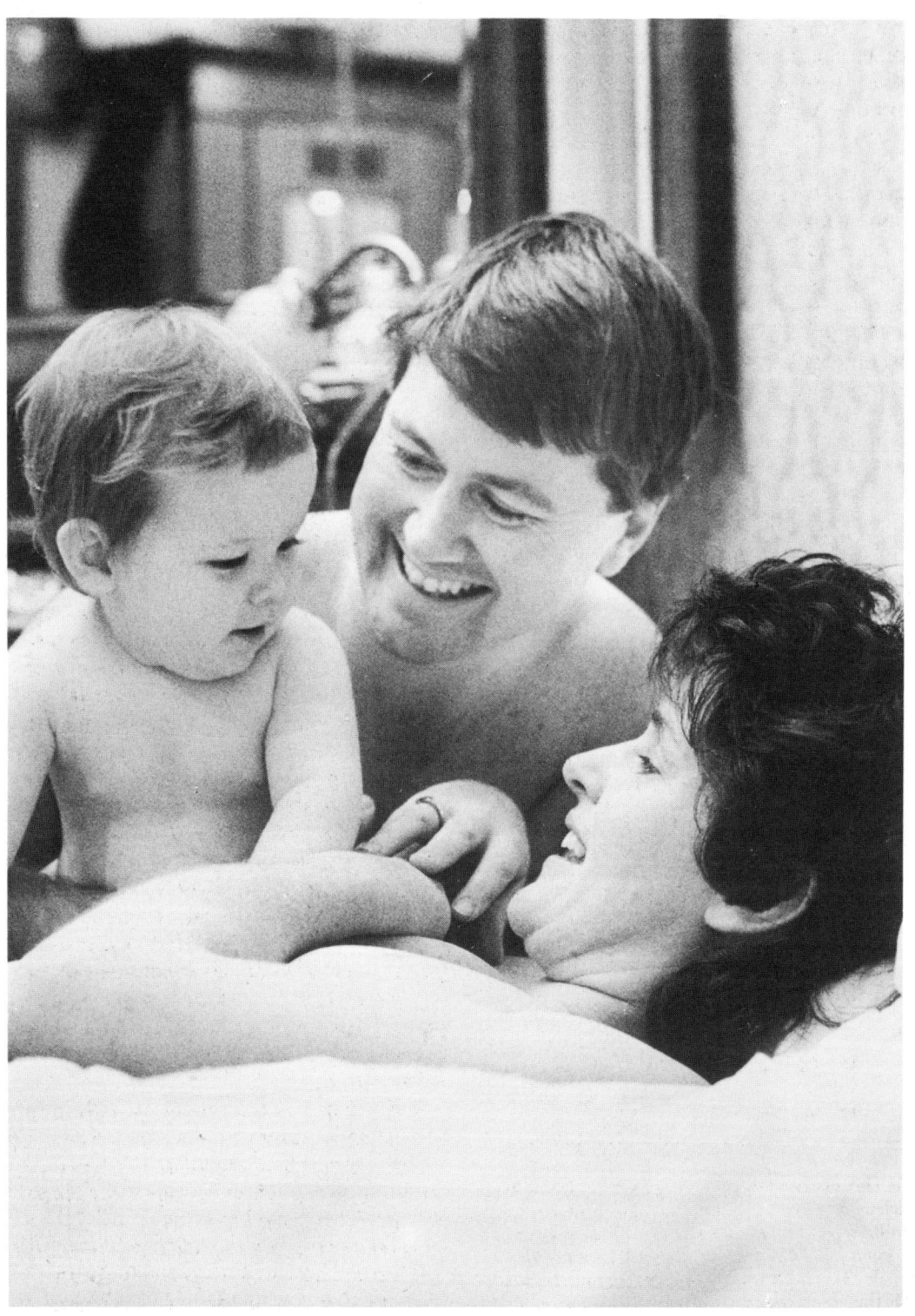

eral chromosomes and one X chromosome. The other half of the spermatozoa have twenty-two general chromosomes and one Y chromosome.

Whether you are male or female depends on whether an X-carrying or a Y-carrying sperm fertilized the ovum your mother made, which developed into you.

If it was a Y-carrying chromosome you will be male; if it was an X-carrying chromosome you will be female.

The gender of a child is determined at the time its father's sperm fertilizes the egg its mother made.

As the **fetus** grows in the mother's uterus, the presence of the Y chromosome in its cells brings about the changes which lead to the development of its **penis** and its **scrotum** containing its testicles. If there is no Y chromosome in the cells, the fetus develops as a female, and instead of a penis a **vagina** is formed.

From birth how you are treated will probably depend on whether you are a boy or a girl, although your parents may be quite unaware that they are treating you differently from how they would treat a child of the opposite gender.

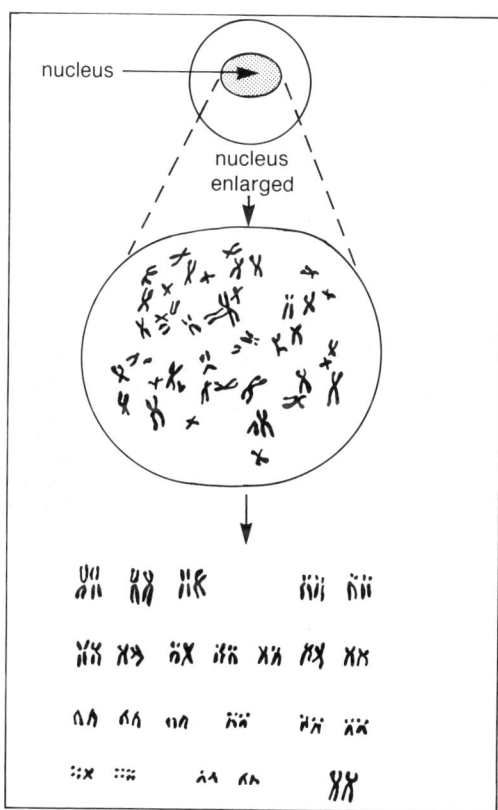

The chromosomes form a tangled skein inside the nucleus of each cell. Using special techniques, they can be separated and displayed in what is called a karyotype. In this diagram the cell came from a female. This is shown by the fact that in the last pair the chromosomes are both X chromosomes

## Learning if you are male or female

As you are probably aware, in our society different types of behaviour are expected from men and women throughout their lives, although these expectations are slowly changing. From the day of our birth we begin to learn that we are male or female, boy or girl, by the way people behave towards us. In the first months of life, in most families, most of the influences come from the mother, and only a few from the father. Mothers behave rather differently to boy babies and to girl babies, and so do fathers. As the child's experience widens, as it becomes aware of more of the objects around it, and as it sees more people, its knowledge of whether it is a boy or a girl is reinforced by these people's behaviour to it.

These experiences encourage a child to behave as its parents and society expect it to. A boy is encouraged to behave in a boyish way. A girl is encouraged to behave as a girl is expected to behave.

In our society, by the age of three a boy has learned how he is expected to behave, so that other people can recognize him as being a boy. Similarly, a girl has learned how she is expected to behave so that people will recognize that she is a girl. In this way boys and girls develop gender roles: that is, they behave as a boy or as a girl is expected to behave.

By the same age, or perhaps a little later, a boy has learned his gender identity, and a girl has learned her gender identity. This means that in most cases a boy has become aware that he is a boy, that he will always be a boy and that he wants to be a boy. In the same way, a girl has most likely become aware that she is a girl, that she doesn't want to be a boy and that she always will be a girl. The gender identity which has been acquired will probably persist throughout life.

A very few children, mostly boys, fail to develop a fixed gender identity. These are the people who grow up convinced that they should belong to the other sex, whatever their anatomy says. They are transsexuals (see chapter 11, p. 102).

In childhood, until puberty, there is very little difference in the physical shape of a boy and a girl apart from the obvious genital difference. But there are obvious differences in their behaviour.

Society teaches boys to be aggressive, to be rough and to be tough. Society discourages boys from being sensitive and gentle. It discourages boys from touching.

On the other hand, society teaches girls to be submissive, gentle, dependent, tidy, clean, helpful and sensitive. It encourages girls to touch and to help others.

The difference in the ways boys and girls behave is not due to their biology—their chromosomes—except to a very small extent. The difference is due to the different way that boys and girls are treated by parents, friends, acquaintances, other children, and by advertising on radio and television. In short, the difference is due to the way that society behaves to boys and girls.

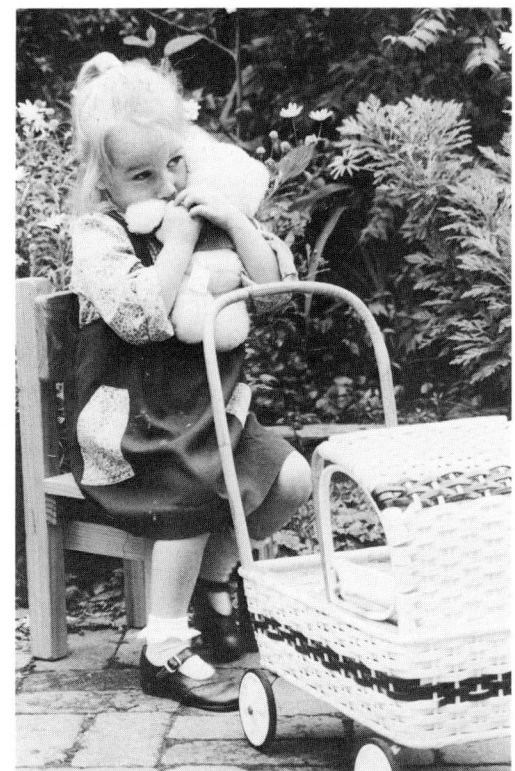

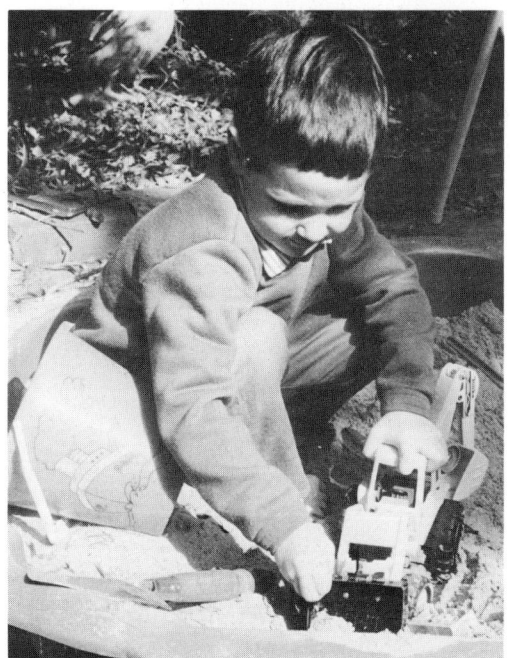

Boys and girls at play in our society

The lessons boys and girls learn of how to behave, of how to fit into their appropriate gender roles, have a considerable effect on the way they behave when they become adults, particularly on the way they behave sexually.

## Sexuality in childhood

Most parents accept, rather reluctantly, that babies are sexual in that they can be seen to enjoy playing with their genitals. Many parents also believe that when the child reaches the age of about three its interest in its sexuality stops. This is not correct. Children play with their genitals at all ages, but because of a widening range of experiences they seem to do it less often after the age of three.

Parents should be aware that the children remain very interested in their sexuality and want to know more about their own sexuality and that of other people (see Box).

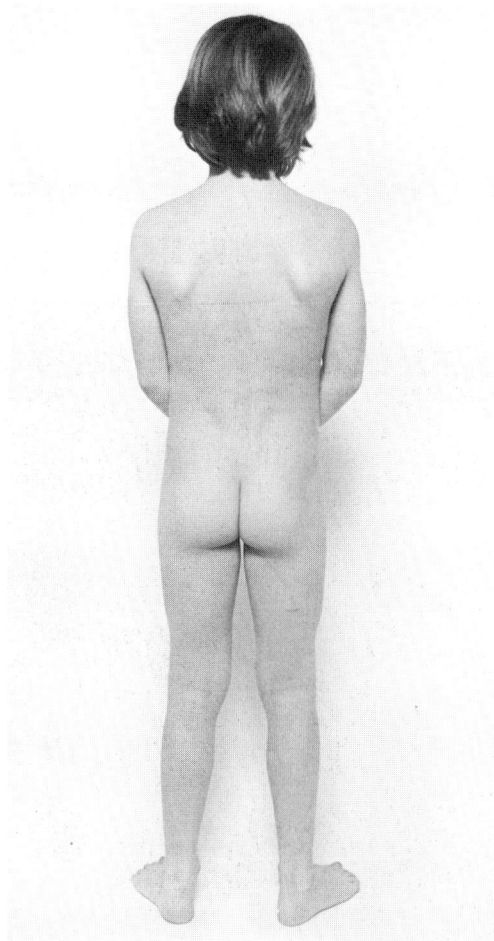
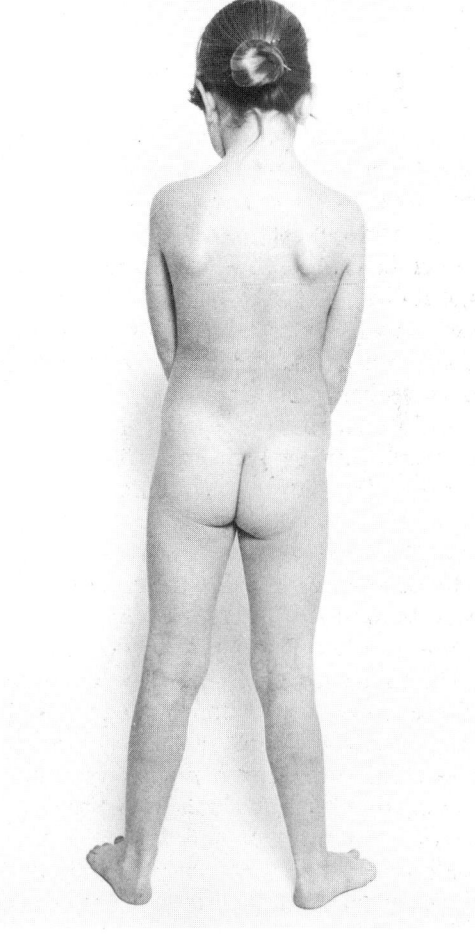

Boy and girl aged 8 years

# Childhood sexuality

| Age of child | General findings | Questions asked |
|---|---|---|
| 3 | Usually knows own sex.<br>Wants to touch its mother's breasts.<br>Plays with its genitals. | Wonders where babies come from. |
| 4 | Under stress holds genitals. | Wonders how babies are born. |
| 5 | Increasing modesty.<br>Aware of sex organs, sex differences. | |
| 6 | Sex play, exhibitionism (at school).<br>Investigates other sex in games like 'mummies and daddies', 'doctors' and 'show me'.<br>Is confused if told by older children about intercourse. | Wonders if giving birth hurts a woman. |
| 7 | Some mutual exploration.<br>Interest in sex role (do what own sex does).<br>Boys and girls usually play separately. | Understands baby is formed from two 'seeds'. |
| 8 | Interest in sex rather high, but exploration decreasing.<br>Interest in 'dirty' words and stories, and 'smutty jokes'. | Girls wonder about menstruation. |
| 9 | Talks about sex with friends.<br>Seeks illustrations about sex.<br>Uses 'sex' swear words.<br>May be self-conscious of naked body. | |

Gesell, A. and Ilg, P. *The Child from Five to Ten*. Harper & Row, N.Y., 1976.

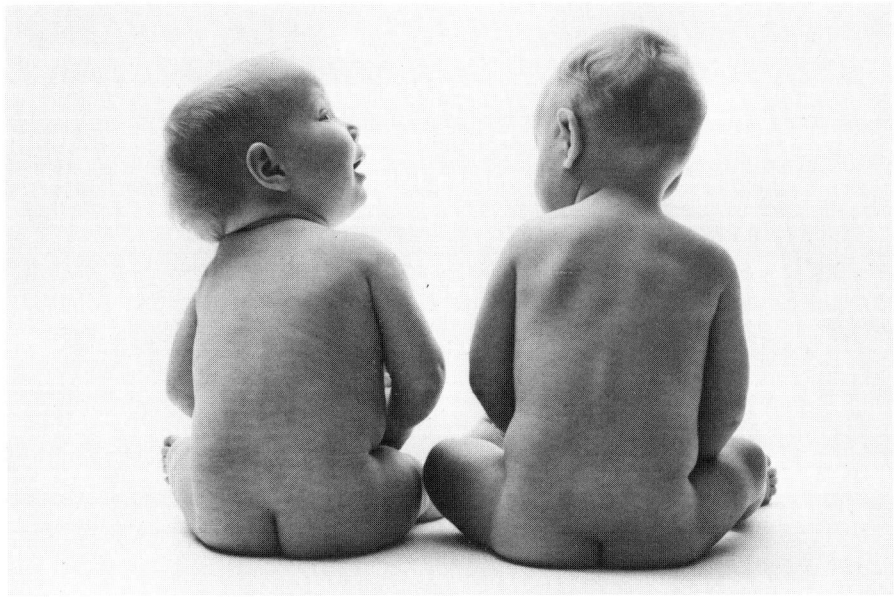

Boy or girl, can you tell?

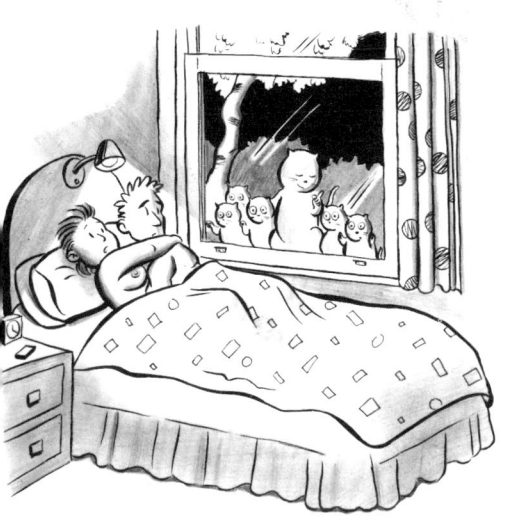

*Investigations*
● Investigate the causes and effects of the expectations that parents and society have of children's behaviour.
● Find out all you can about the stages of physical development which a child will go through in the first six years of life.

*Discussions*
● Think of some examples of particular ways in which parents, and society in general, expect children of different sexes to behave.
● Discuss the ways (apart from sexual intercourse) in which people express themselves sexually.

*Activities*
● Write down your thoughts and feelings about your own sexuality and discuss them with others in your group and, if possible, with your friends and family.

# 2
# YOUR SEXUAL ORGANS: FEMALE AND MALE

You can't really understand human sexuality unless you know something about your sexual organs. Males usually know more about them because the main sexual organs of a man are outside his body, easily visible and easy to touch. A woman's sexual organs are mostly inside her body. Many women, it seems, have never looked between their legs to see the sexual organs which are on the outside of their bodies, nor have they ever touched them with a clear knowledge of what it is they are touching.

## A woman's sexual organs

The anatomical name for a woman's external sexual organs is the **vulva**. The name used by many people when trying to speak about the vulva is the private parts, although shorter words are used privately (see Glossary). The vulva comprises several structures and tissues which surround the entrance to the **vagina**, which is the hollow tube leading to a woman's uterus.

Each of the tissues of the vulva has its own separate function. Furthest out from the vaginal entrance, the **large lips** (the **labia majora**), are two large, soft folds of skin under which there are pads of fatty tissue. The skin of the lips has hair on its outer surface and sweat glands on its inner surface. In front (looked at from between the woman's legs) the two large lips form a pad of fat which lies on the pubic bone. Because the lips and the fat pad in front are most developed in the years when a woman is most active sexually, the fat pad is called the **mount of Venus**. The mount is covered with curly hair in a woman whose body has gone through the changes of puberty. The amount of hair varies. Some women have a great deal; in other women the hair is scanty. Both are normal. The pubic hair ends on the upper side of the mount in a straight line in women (men have pubic hair which extends up to the **umbilicus** [belly button] as an upside down V). When a woman has her legs together the large lips lie close to each other and conceal the inner vulva. When her legs are apart the inner vulva can be seen.

The inner surface of the big lips is separated by a narrow groove from the delicate **small lips** (or **labia minora**). The small lips are folds of delicate skin, and vary in size quite considerably. Some women have long lips, in other women the lips are small. It used to be thought that large lips were due to masturbation, but this is now known to be untrue.

In front the two lips join, splitting into two folds, one of which goes above and the other below the **clitoris**. The clitoris is the equivalent of a man's penis. It is a small pinkish nob, the size of a pea. It is composed of tissue which fills with blood when a woman is aroused sexually. It is very sensitive to touch; if a woman fondles her clitoris with her finger, or if it is caressed by her partner, she may have an orgasm. During sexual intercourse her clitoris is also stimulated, although indirectly, by the movement of the man's penis in her vagina.

Most women have never used a mirror to look at their clitoris. It is something every woman should do, so that she knows what her vulva looks like; and she should then touch the parts to feel their textures.

The area below the clitoris and between the small lips is called the **entrance**, or **vestibule**, to the vagina. Just below the clitoris is the external opening of the **urinary tract** (the **urethra**).

Below the urethra, the **hymen** (or **maidenhead**) surrounds the vaginal entrance. The hymen is a thin, incomplete fold of membrane with one or more gaps in it. It varies very considerably in shape and elasticity. When a woman has sexual intercourse for the first time, the hymen is stretched or torn slightly. If it is torn, a small amount of bleeding may occur. In many cultures, the tearing of the hymen and the bleeding was considered a sign that the girl was a virgin at the time of her marriage. The bed was inspected on the morning after the first night of the honeymoon for the evidence of blood. An 'intact' hymen is not a reliable sign of virginity, as it may have been stretched previously, by the exploring fingers of the girl herself or by her partner during heavy petting.

Beneath the hymen, deep in the soft tissues of the vulva, two pea-sized glands called **Bartholin's glands** are connected by ducts to the vagina. When a woman is sexually excited these glands add moisture to the vaginal entrance.

The part of the vulva between the vagina and the rectum is made up of muscles. It is called the **perineum** and is of great importance during childbirth, when it has to stretch so that the baby can be born.

The rest of a woman's genital organs are inside her body.

The **vagina** is a hollow tube lined with soft 'velvety' cells. It is surrounded by muscles and stretches upwards and backwards from the entrance to reach the uterus. Normally its walls lie close together and are only separated by a penis during sexual intercourse, the insertion of some

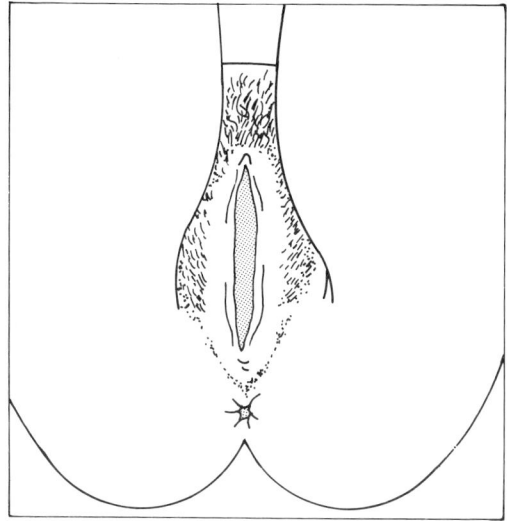

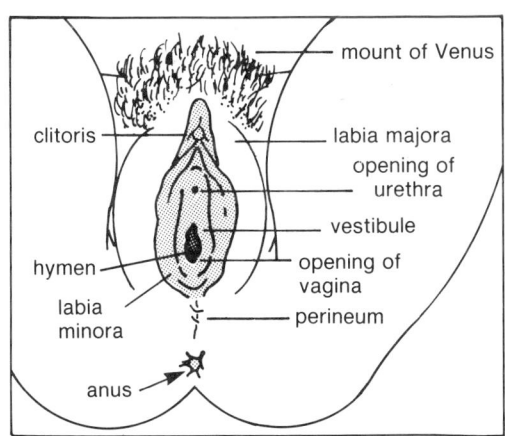

The vulval region. When a woman's legs are together only the labia majora are seen. They hide all the other parts of the vulva. When a woman opens her legs, the details of the vulval structures can be seen

objects such as a tampon during menstruation, a finger touching and exploring, or a baby being born. You can understand from this that the vagina can expand easily and it is never too small for sexual intercourse. A woman who finds intercourse painful is not 'small-made'. She is resisting intercourse because fear, anxiety or embarrassment make her tighten the muscles which surround her vagina.

The vagina is a remarkable organ. It is capable of great expansion and it keeps itself clean and healthy. The cells which line the vagina lie on top of each other like a wall of bricks, thirty cells thick. During a woman's reproductive years (from about the age of fourteen to fifty-four), the top layer of cells is constantly being shed into the vagina. The cells which are shed interact with a small bacillus (or germ) which lives in the vagina to produce a substance called lactic acid. Lactic acid helps to keep a woman's vagina clean and healthy.

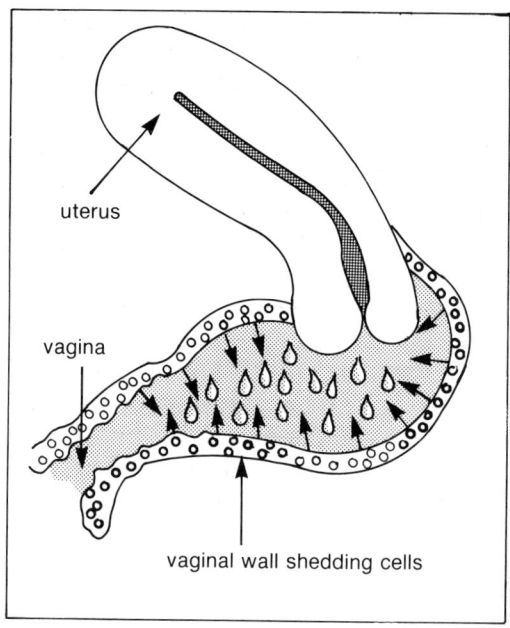

Vaginal cells 'exfoliating' into the vagina to produce lactic acid, which keeps the vagina clean and healthy

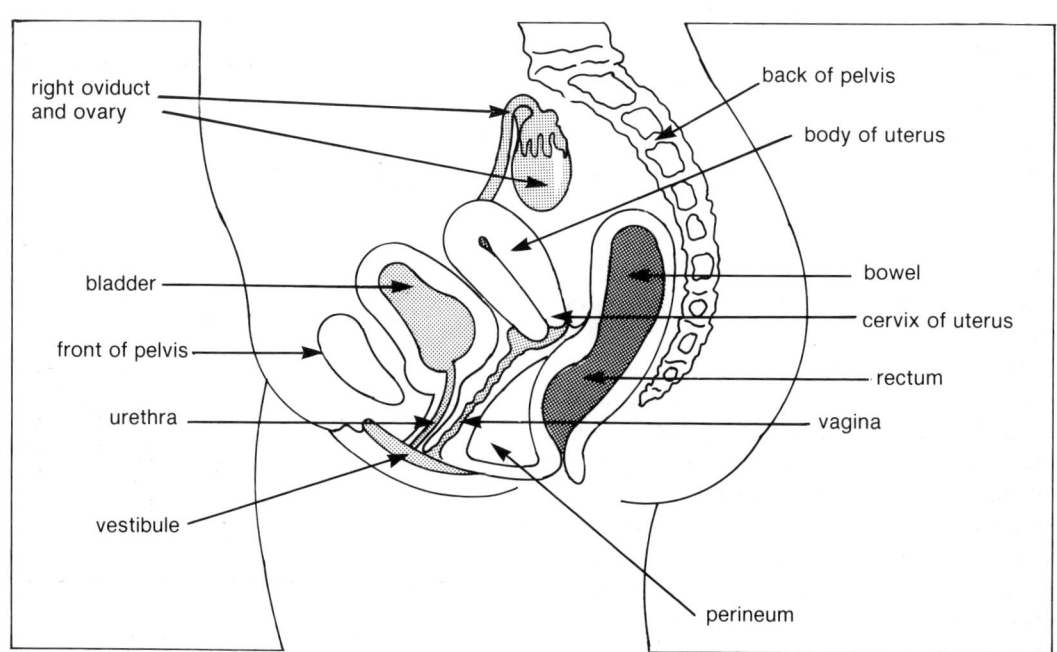

The internal genital organs of a woman

The **cervix**, or **neck** of the **uterus**, pokes into the upper part of the vagina. The cervix is a place where cancer may develop, usually when a woman is in her forties or fifties. Nobody knows why cancer should develop there, but it may be due to genital wart virus infection many years earlier. Nuns rarely get cancer of the cervix, and prostitutes often do, so it is related in some way to sexual intercourse. One theory is that sexual intercourse with several partners before the age of 25 may be an important factor because of the increased chance that one of them will have wart virus infection of his penis, although the warts may be so small they cannot be seen. Doctors recommend that sexually active women have cancer tests (called Pap smears) made at intervals, although cervical cancer is rare in young women and only affects two in every hundred older women.

The Pap smear test is made by gently introducing a small metal instrument into the vagina. It is called a speculum and looks like a duck's beak. When the beak is opened the doctor can see the cervix. The cervix is stroked (rubbed gently) with a flat piece of wood, the size of a pencil, called a spatula. This causes some of the cells which cover the cervix to stick to the spatula. They are then smeared onto a glass slide and looked at through a microscope. Some smears reveal abnormal cells which may lead, if not treated, to cancer some years later.

The Pap smear is a painless test and a woman who is sexually active should have the test made twice in the first year she has sex, and then every one to three years throughout her life. You can get a test done on your cervix if you go along to your local Family Planning Clinic or to your doctor.

Above the cervix, the main part of the **uterus** or **womb** (called the **corpus** or **body**), looks like a small pear held so that the neck points downwards. The uterus is a

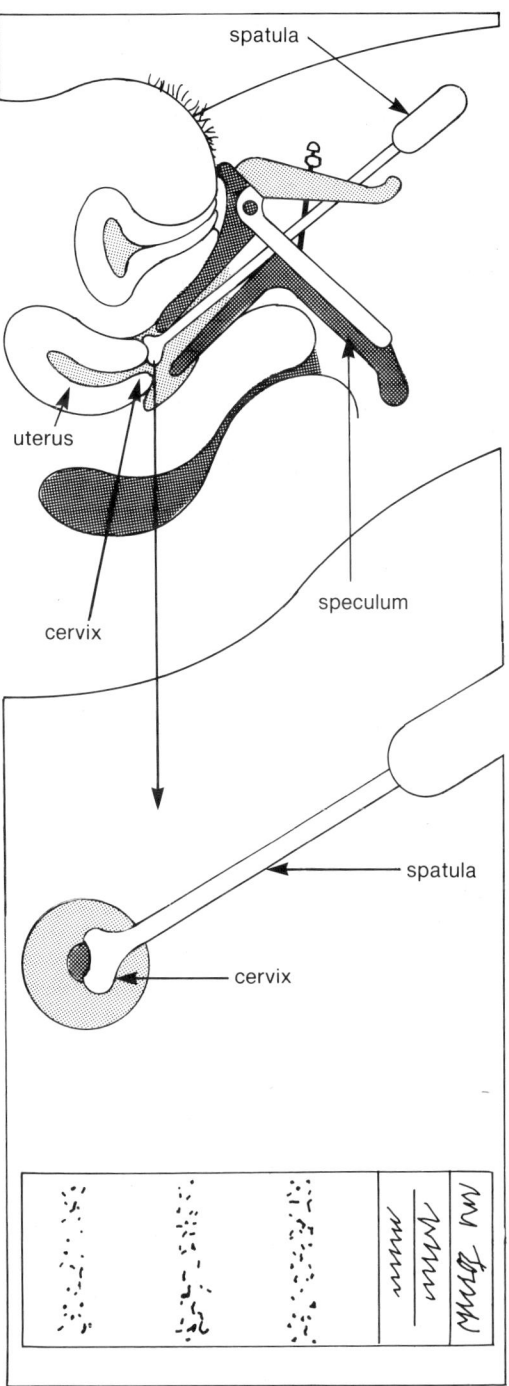

How a Pap smear is taken. Although it looks complicated, it is not, and it is painless if the doctor is experienced and gentle

11

hollow muscular organ which lies in the centre of the bony pelvis, between the bladder and the bowel. It is about 9 cm long and weighs nearly 60 g. During pregnancy, the uterus grows considerably and stretches. By the time the baby is due to be born it is about 45 cm long and weighs 1000 g.

Normally the inner walls of the uterus are close to each other so that its cavity is slit-like and triangular in shape. The cavity is lined with special cells and glands called the **endometrium**. Most of the endometrium crumbles away and is discharged from the uterus, mixed with a small amount of blood and a larger quantity of tissue fluid when a woman has a menstrual period.

Usually the uterus is bent forward at an angle of 90 degrees, and rests against the bladder. As the bladder fills with urine the uterus rotates backwards; as the bladder empties the uterus falls forward. In about ten per cent of women, the uterus lies bent backwards. This is called a retroversion. In the past a retroversion was considered to be a serious condition which caused sterility, backache and many other complaints. Today it is known that a retroverted uterus is usually normal and rarely causes any trouble.

The **oviducts** (or **Fallopian tubes**) are two narrow tubes, one on each side of the uterus, which stretch for about 10 cm from its upper angles to lie in contact with the ovaries. The outer end of each tube is divided into long finger-like processes which sweep up the egg when it is pushed out from the **ovary**. The oviducts are of great importance. In their outer portion the egg

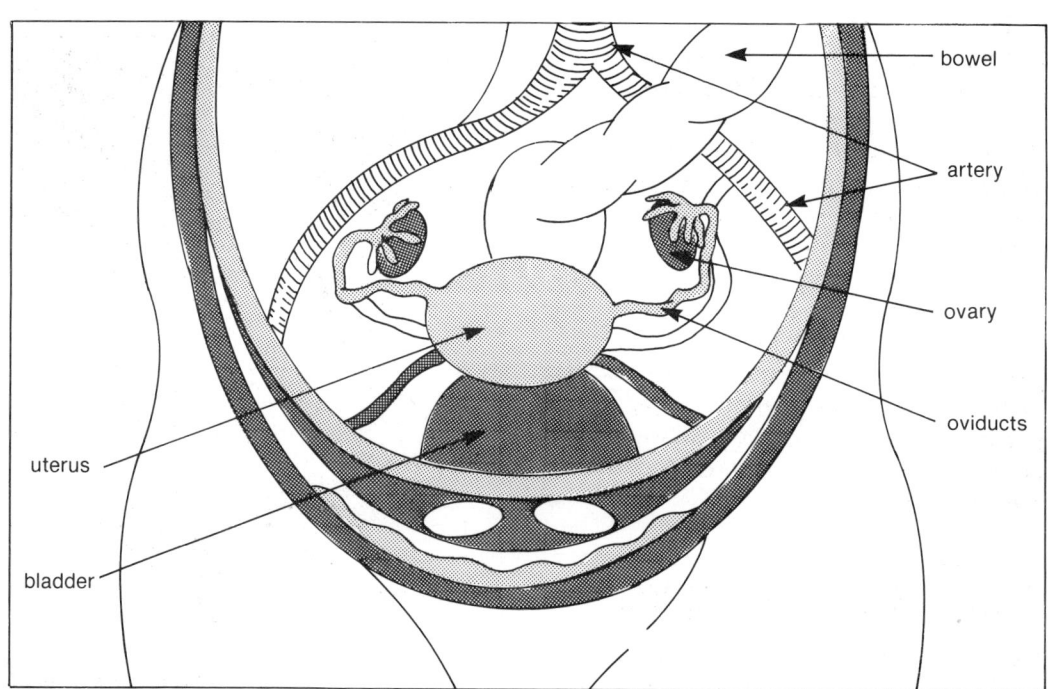

bowel

artery

ovary

oviducts

uterus

bladder

At operation when a surgeon opens the abdomen he sees the uterus, the oviducts and the tubes lying between the bladder and the bowel

12

is fertilized by the sperm and pregnancy begins. Some of the cells lining the oviducts provide nourishment for the fertilized egg; other cells have long fronds, like seagrass, which gently move the fertilized egg towards the cavity of the uterus. The oviducts can be damaged by infections, especially chlamydial infection and gonorrhoea (see p. 92) and then the woman may be unable to have any children.

The **ovaries** are two oval-shaped organs, which each contain over 200 000 tiny round cells. Any one of these primitive cells can become an ovum, or egg, if it is stimulated by the appropriate hormone from the brain. The egg cells are surrounded by a meshwork of supporting tissue which makes up most of the ovary. Each month, from puberty to about the age of fifty, about twenty cells are stimulated to grow, but only one of them develops sufficiently to become an ovum.

The ovary is also an important hormone factory. Hormones are substances which are released into the blood stream and which act on other tissues. Hormones produced in the brain reach the ovaries by way of the blood and stimulate them to produce the female sex hormones oestrogen and progesterone. At puberty the effect of these hormones is to make a woman's breasts grow and her hips become rounder. Each month from puberty until a woman reaches the menopause or 'change of life' the hormones prepare her body, particularly the uterus, for a pregnancy. If no pregnancy occurs, the woman has a menstrual period.

# A man's sexual organs

Most of a man's sexual organs are outside the body. His external genital organs consist of his **penis** and his two **testicles**, which lie in his scrotum between his legs, below the root of his penis.

Normally, unless a man is sexually aroused, his penis is soft and limp and hangs down slackly. The size of a man's unstimulated penis varies a good deal. Some men have small penises, measuring 6 cm in length. Other men have penises measuring 16 cm in length. The circumference of the penis also varies a good deal. When a man is sexually aroused his penis becomes erect—it fills with blood and becomes stiff and points upwards. During erection, a small penis grows more than a large penis, so the difference in length of erect penises is not great.

Anyway, a big penis doesn't make a man a better lover; that depends on his appreciation of his partner's needs and desires, and on the way he relates to his partner.

If a man has not been circumcised, his foreskin peels back slightly when his penis

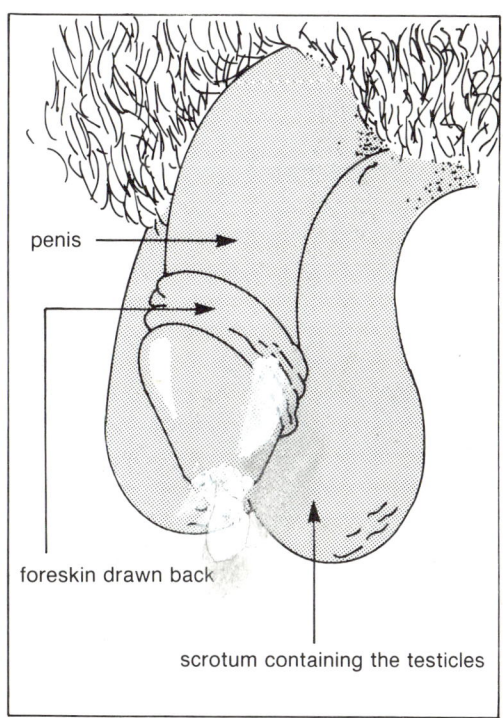

penis

foreskin drawn back

scrotum containing the testicles

The external genitals of a man

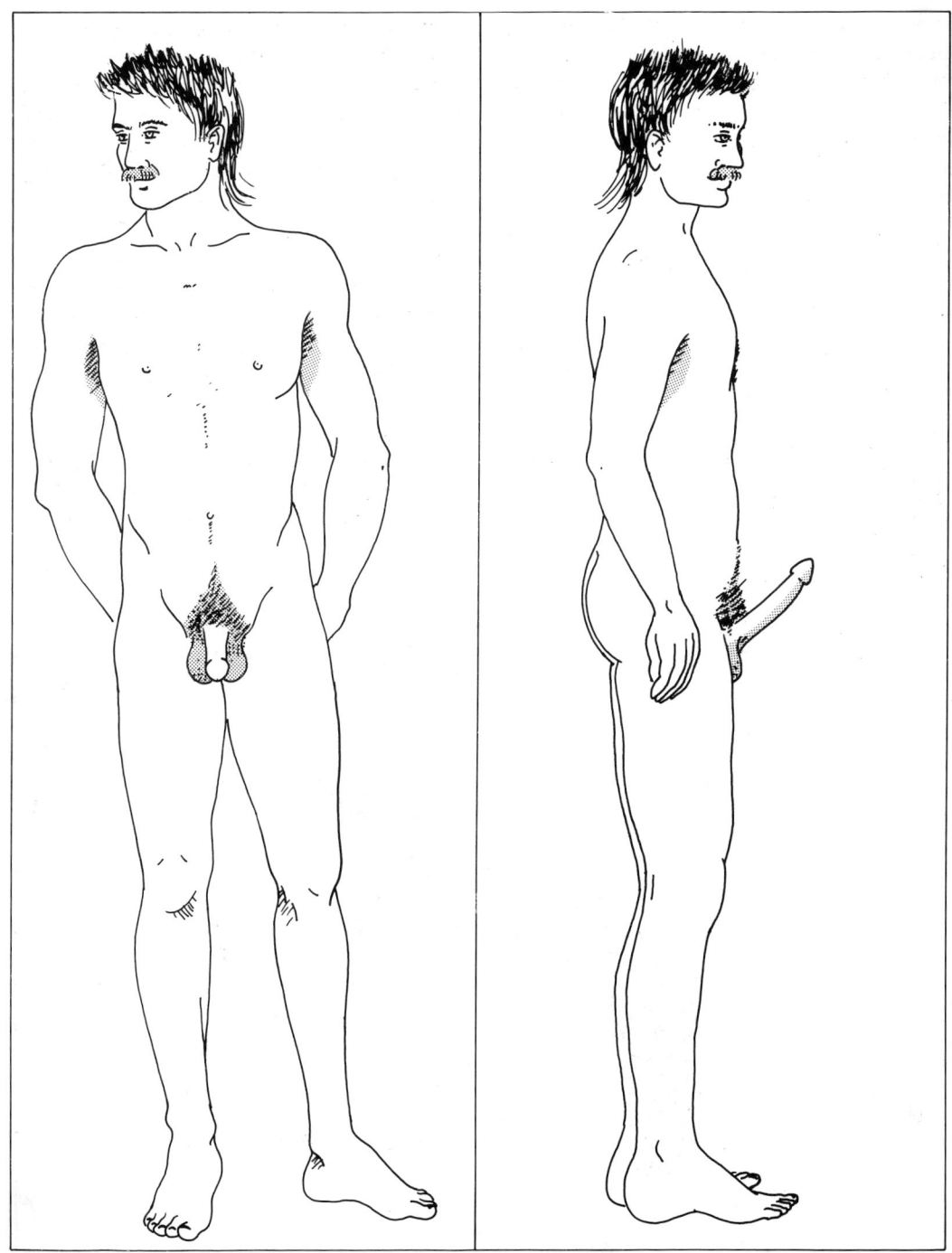

The external genital organs of a man with a
flaccid, non-stimulated penis and with an erect,
stimulated penis

is erect, to expose part of the head of the penis, which is called the **glans**. If he pulls his foreskin fully back the whole glans is exposed. The glans is covered with a delicate mucous membrane (similar to that inside your cheeks) which is very sensitive to touch. During sexual intercourse a man's foreskin peels back fully so that the entire glans and the shaft of the penis are stimulated as the man thrusts forwards and backwards inside the woman's soft, wet vagina.

On the under surface of the penis a band of tissue, called the **frenulum**, stops the foreskin from being drawn too far back. The frenulum starts just behind the opening of the man's urethra, the 'eye' of his penis, and runs back in a small cleft in the glans.

Removal of the foreskin, or circumcision, is performed in certain cultures for ritual reasons when the boy is a baby (for example amongst the Jewish people), or at puberty to mark manhood (for example, amongst the Arab people and others of the Islamic faith). In modern times, in Australia and the USA particularly, circumcision is done, not for religious reasons, but because it has become the usual thing to do.

Increasing numbers of parents today, however, are deciding not to have their boy babies circumcised. One advantage of this is that the foreskin protects the delicate glans of the penis from damage. Circumcision does not stop a boy masturbating. Circumcision does not make a man last longer before reaching orgasm during sexual

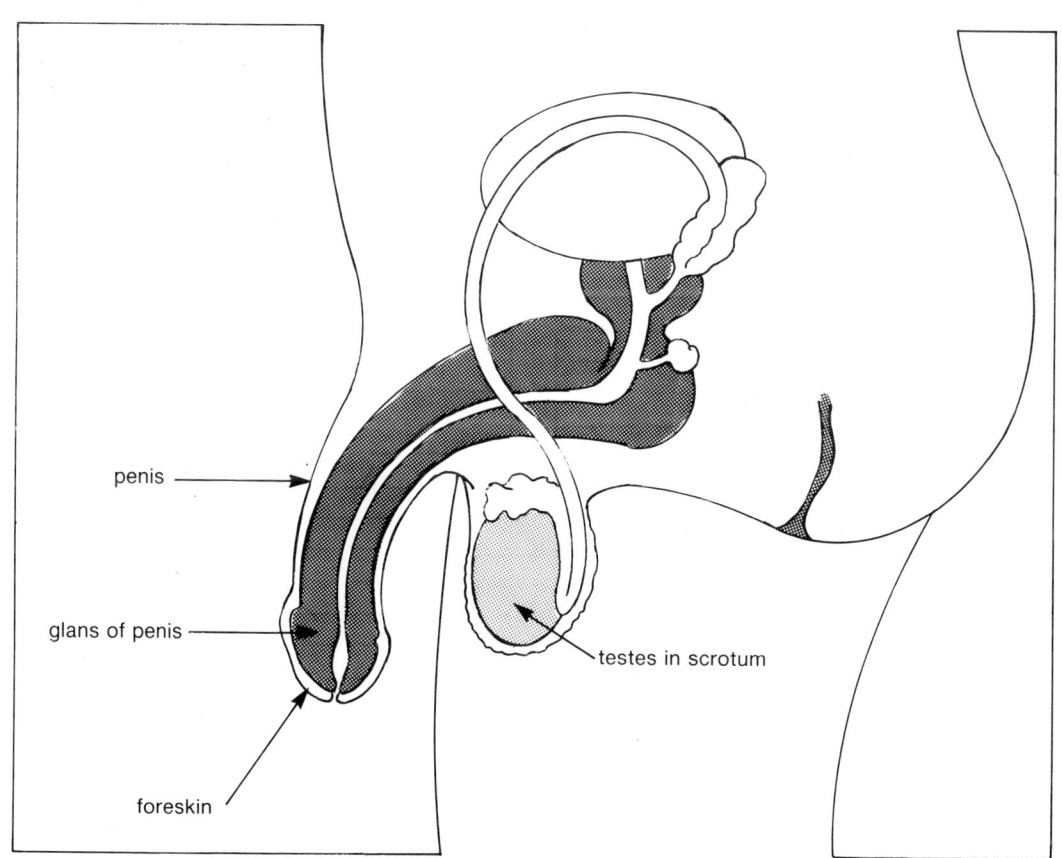

penis

glans of penis

foreskin

testes in scrotum

Internal and external genital organs of a man

intercourse. Circumcision does not encourage hygiene. If an uncircumcised man draws back the foreskin and washes his glans he is as clean as a circumcised man.

The tube connecting the bladder to the body surface passes through the penis, ending at the eye of the penis. It is called the **urethra**.

The urethra is longer in a man than in a woman. It is S-shaped and extends along the under surface of the penis, through the prostate gland, to reach the bladder. It has two functions. You pass urine through it, and sperms also pass through it to be ejaculated at orgasm.

The **prostate gland** is shaped like a chestnut and lies below the bladder, deep inside a man's pelvis. The urethra passes through it, as do two other hollow tubes. These are the two vasa deferentia (singular: **vas deferens**). These tubes reach from the testes to join each other and the urethra within the substance of the prostate gland. Sperms formed in the testes pass along the vasa on their way to be ejaculated when a man has an orgasm. Just before the vasa enter the substance of the prostate they become wider and two closed pouches form, called **seminal vesicles**.

The vasa enable sperm to travel from the

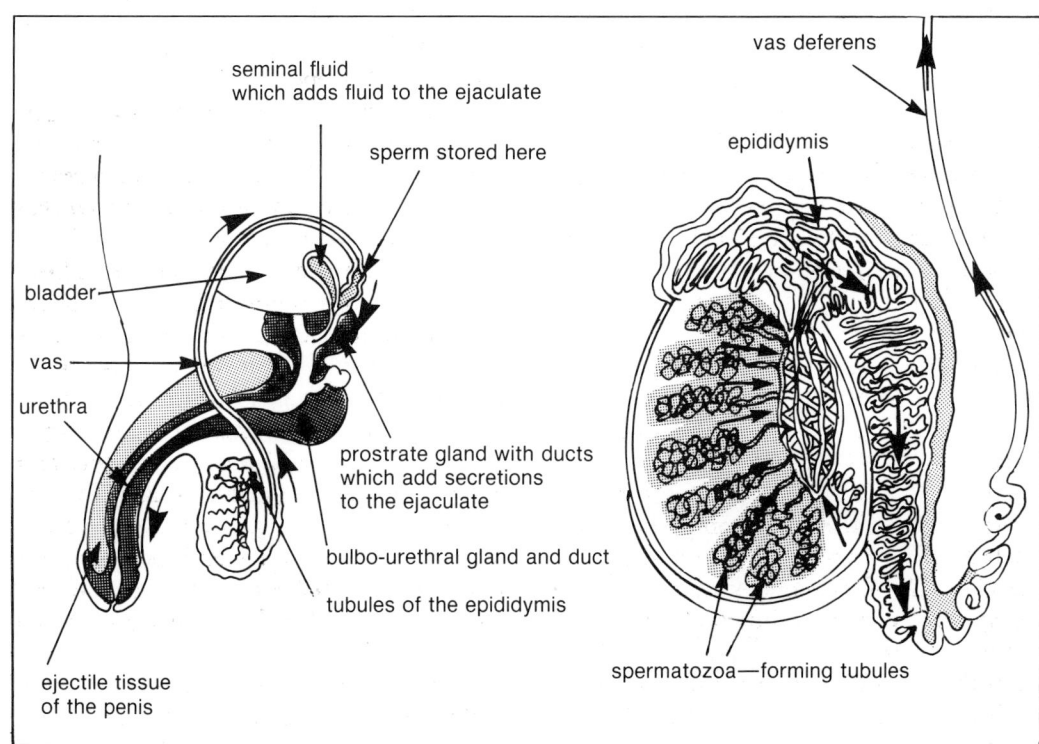

The journey of the sperm from its formation in the testes to its ejaculation is shown by the arrows. The sperm producing tubules in the testes are shown in greater detail

testicles, where they are formed, to reach the distended part (the seminal vesicles) where they are stored, ready for ejaculation. The seminal vesicles provide nourishment for the sperms.

A man can feel his vas if he holds his scrotum between a finger and thumb where it joins his body. If you roll the tissues between your finger and thumb you will detect a cord-like structure—that is the vas.

Each vas begins in a long twisted narrow tube, like a tangled bundle of string, which lies alongside the surface of the testicle, like a cockscomb. This is called the **epididymis**, and in it sperms mature.

The epididymis connects with the vas at one end and at the other with the narrow tubes which make up most of the testicle.

The **testicles**, or **testes**, are smooth oval structures which are very tender if squeezed, and which lie one in each side of the scrotum. Each testicle is made up of about 250 small segments, like the sections of an orange. Each segment is made up of a twisted tube lined with cells.

The sperm are formed in the cell nests at the rate of 50 000 every minute, from puberty into old age. They go through several changes as they develop. Then they are shed into the hollow tubes of the segments of the testes and slowly move along the twisted tubes of the epididymis, and enter the vas. They move along the vas to reach the storage area in the prostate gland. They reach maturity only when they reach the dilated part of the vas in the prostate gland. It takes 80 days from the time the sperms start forming until they are mature and ready to be ejaculated. Only when the sperm is mature is it capable of fertilizing the egg (ovum) to create a new human being.

The testicles are also hormone factories. From about the age of twelve, they produce the male sex hormone **testosterone**. They will go on doing this into very old age, although the peak production of testosterone is between the ages of twenty and forty-five.

Testosterone is the main hormone which turns a boy into a man, as you will find out in the next chapter. It makes his genital organs grow, from the age of twelve or thereabouts, so that his penis reaches its adult size by the age of sixteen. Some boys mature sexually early, some don't become sexually mature until later. Both are normal.

Testosterone has several other effects. It enlarges a man's voice box so that his voice changes, eventually 'breaking' when it becomes more gruff. During the time of change a boy is less well able to control the range of his voice. He may start a sentence hoarsely only to find that halfway through he starts 'squeaking'. It can be embarrassing, but it is normal for this to happen during adolescence.

Testosterone is responsible for triggering the growth of hair on a man's and on a woman's body. The hair grows on a man's face, on his pubis, in his armpits and on his chest. Some men have a lot of facial and body hair. Some men have very little. Both have the same amount of testosterone circulating in their blood, but a man who has little body hair has hair follicles which are rather insensitive to testosterone. It does not mean that there is anything wrong.

The hair on a woman's body, especially around her vulva, over the mount of Venus and in the armpits, grows because of testosterone circulating in her blood. Women make very much less testosterone and consequently grow much less body or facial hair.

Testosterone is also responsible for making the sweat glands in the skin more active. The sweat glands produce a grease called sebum which keeps the skin soft and supple. If the glands become over-active the nature of the grease changes. Instead of being a thin lubricant, it becomes thick and

# Circumcision

| Myth | Reality |
|------|---------|
| • It makes the penis cleaner and prevents disease. | • Untrue. The penis is only likely to be dirty if a man fails to draw back his foreskin and wash his glans when he showers or bathes. |
| • It discourages masturbation. | • It doesn't. Most men masturbate by stimulating the shaft of their penis, not the glans. |
| • It delays a man's orgasm. | • It doesn't. |
| • It prevents cancer of the cervix developing in the man's wife. | • This was once believed but has now been shown to be untrue. |
| • It prevents cancer of the penis. | • This is possible, but if a man washes his penis regularly after drawing back the foreskin, cancer of the penis is unlikely. It is a very rare cancer. |

sticky. Sometimes the thicker grease cannot escape from the gland and a blackhead or a whitehead forms. If germs get into the blocked gland, a painful infected pimple may form. If there are many infected sweat glands the result is acne, which is common amongst teenagers.

Acne has nothing to do with dirtiness, although washing regularly with soap and water helps remove the thick sebum. Acne is not caused by constipation, too many sweet foods, or by masturbation. Mild, non-disfiguring acne generally responds to medications applied to the skin, or to taking oral contraceptives. More severe acne, particularly if it is lumpy or if scarring is occurring, needs other treatment, which can only be prescribed by a doctor as the drugs, although effective, may cause side-effects.

*Investigations*
• Investigate some of the customs present in our culture and in other cultures concerning circumcision.
• What are some of the beliefs upheld in our society with respect to the hymen and vaginal discharges? See if you can find any information about comparable beliefs in other societies.

*Discussions*
• Discuss some of the myths associated with sexual performance (e.g. a big penis makes a man a good lover).
• Discuss some of the advantages and disadvantages of circumcision.

*Activities*
• Find objects of similar size and shape to the uterus and the ovaries.
• List as many words as you can which can be used for penis, vagina, vulva. Can they be categorized according to sex, age, culture of those who use them?
• If you are female, use a mirror to identify your vagina, clitoris, labia majora and labia minora.

# 3
# PUBERTY, ADOLESCENCE AND SEXUALITY

Puberty is a period of change. Puberty is a period of growth and development, particularly of a person's sexuality. It is a period when the hormones secreted by the **pituitary gland** at the base of the brain begin to circulate in the blood in increasing amounts.

These hormones act on the sex glands (the testes and the ovaries) and cause them to release increasing amounts of sex hormones. These sex hormones, in turn, cause boys' and girls' bodies to develop differently.

Puberty is a process. It takes time for a person to come to full physical and sexual maturity. It is also an event marked by definite changes in the bodies of girls and boys. At the onset of puberty a girl first menstruates and becomes capable of conceiving a baby. It is the time a boy first ejaculates sperm and is capable of fathering a baby. Puberty merges imperceptibly into adolescence.

Adolescence is the period during which a child is in the process of becoming a mature person—physically, mentally, emotionally, socially. When adolescence ends —around the early twenties, although there is no clearly defined time—the person is then considered to be an adult. The process of changing and becoming more mature is an ongoing one which continues throughout one's life.

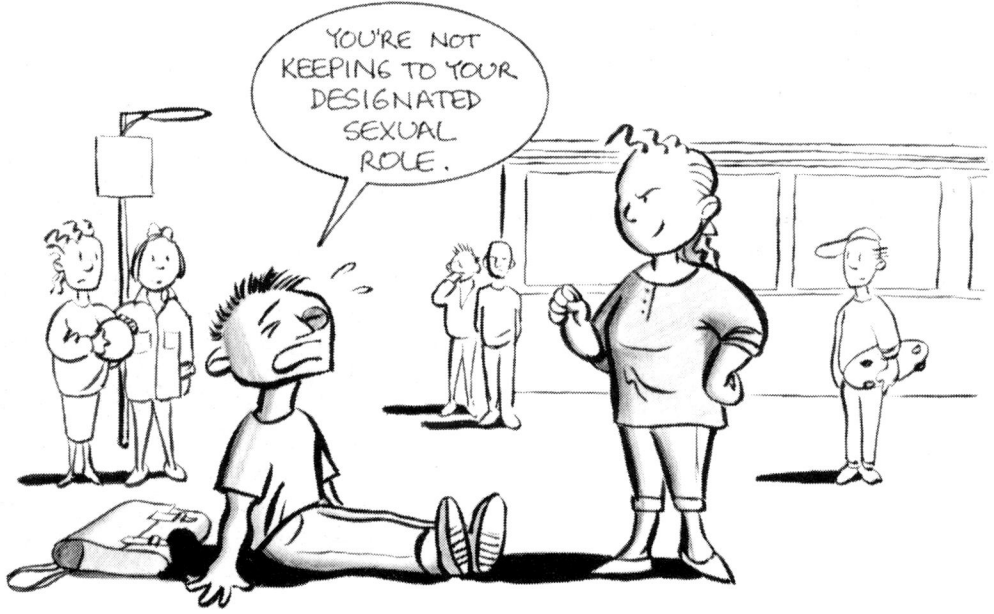

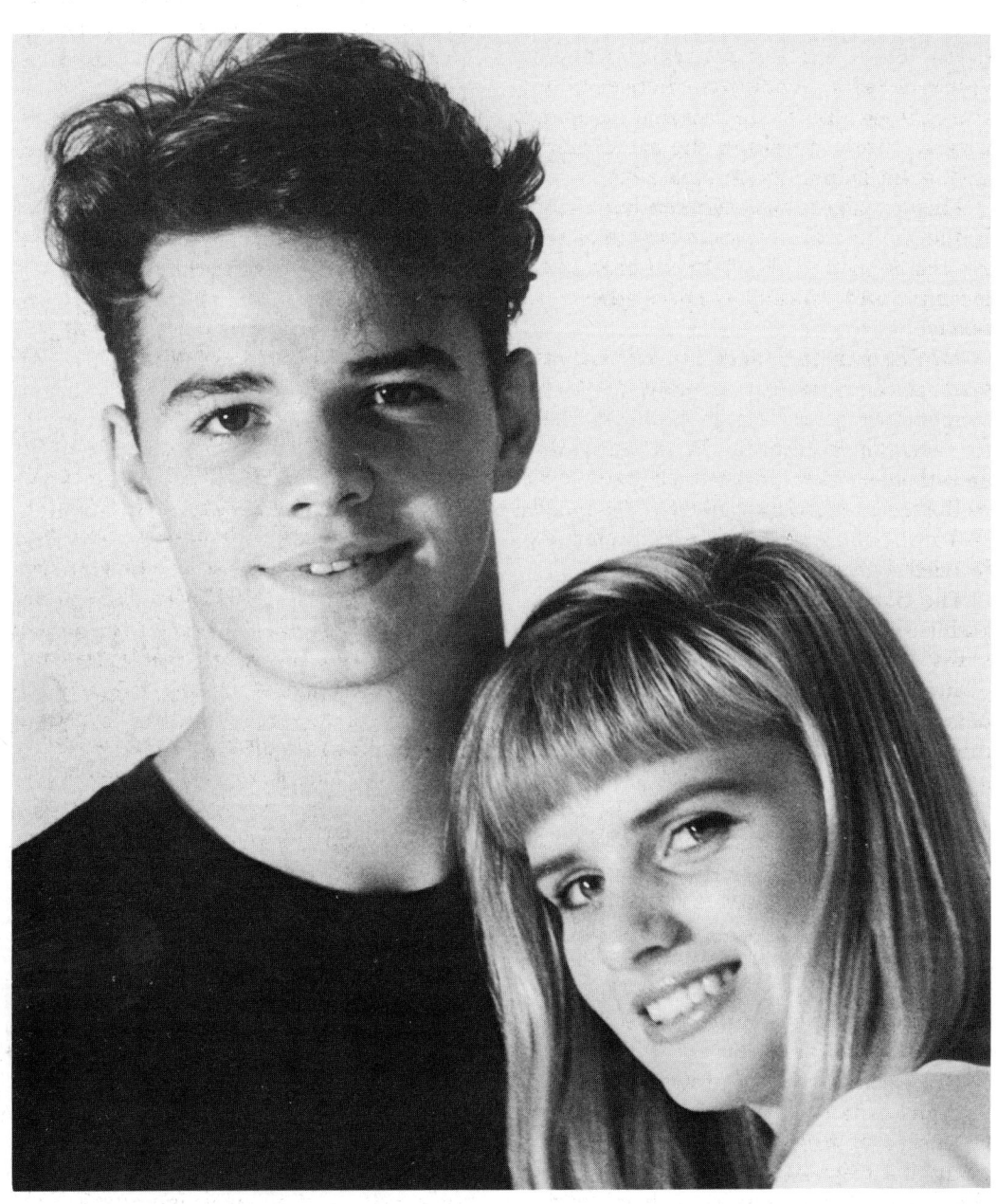

# Puberty and body growth

Up to the age of about nine or ten, there is very little physical difference between boys and girls, except for the fact that a boy has a penis. Both are about the same height and, from behind, both look alike.

They usually behave differently, but that is due to the different ways boys and girls are reared and to the different ways their parents and society expect them to behave.

At about the age of ten or eleven, girls start growing faster and put on more weight than boys. This growth spurt lasts for about three years. Boys start their growth spurt later (about the age of twelve or thirteen) but it lasts longer, so that boys end up, when men, by being taller and heavier than women.

The time the growth spurt starts varies within the sexes, as well as between the sexes. Some boys and girls begin their growth spurt at eleven, in some it is delayed until the age of fifteen. The 'late maturers' often feel embarrassed; so do some early maturers.

The growth spurt is due to a hormone which is released into the blood by the pituitary gland which lies beneath the brain. The first parts of the body to grow are the hands and feet, followed by the hips and chest. The trunk increases in length and the chest deepens. The deepening chest may be hidden in a girl because her breasts are also growing.

During the period of growth spurt, boys and girls often feel and look awkward.

During this time, too, sex differences in body shape become obvious. Because of the female sex hormones in her blood, a girl's hips grow more quickly than her shoulders, and her pelvis becomes wider, rounder and more shallow than that of a boy. Fat is laid down on her hips and she begins to develop a female shape.

A boy's shoulder bones grow more quickly than his pelvis, becoming wider and heavier, and, because of the male sex hormones in his blood, he begins to develop a masculine shape.

These changes occur because sex hormones, in addition to the growth hormone, are now circulating in the blood. As well as altering the body appearance of the two sexes so greatly, these sex hormones make a person's genital organs grow.

# Puberty and sexual development

Why does the development of a person's sexual characteristics begin at puberty? The trigger is the release of hormones, called **gonadotrophins**, by the pituitary gland at the base of the brain. The gonadotrophins stimulate a boy's testes and a girl's ovaries to produce the sex hormones, which then enter the blood stream. The testicles produce the male sex hormone **testosterone** and a small amount of the female sex hormone **oestrogren**. The ovaries produce three hormones. These are **oestrogen**, a second female sex hormone called **progesterone**, and a small amount of **testosterone**.

In females the gonadotrophins also lead to the growth of the egg-cells in the ovaries, and in males they control the production of sperms in the testes.

As we have already seen, the sex hormones help in producing the changes in the shape of a boy's or a girl's body. They also stimulate the growth of the male and female sex organs. Testosterone makes a boy's testes and his penis increase in size. Oestrogen helps a girl's vagina and uterus grow and causes her breasts to develop. In both sexes, testosterone makes hair grow in the armpits, on the lower abdomen and around the genitals.

# What the sex hormones do to your body

## Oestrogen

- Enlarges a girl's breasts.
- Helps deposit fat on her hips
- Makes her vagina, her uterus and her oviducts grow.
- Makes her vagina moist and helps keep it 'clean'.
- Triggers sexual arousal, desire and urge in females.

## Testosterone

- Puts hair on a boy's face and his body, and on the pubis of both boys and girls.
- Increases the muscle mass and strength of males.
- Makes a boy's penis and his testicles grow.
- Enlarges a boy's 'voice box' so that his voice breaks.
- Stimulates a boy's sweat-glands and is a factor in causing adolescent acne.
- Triggers sexual desire, arousal and urge in males.

The age at which these changes occur varies considerably from person to person. Some boys grow tall, get a male body shape, and start getting a bigger penis at twelve or thirteen, in others the growth does not start until fifteen or sixteen. A similar variation in sexual development occurs amongst girls. In some girls sexual maturity comes early. In others the development of the breasts starts later and the growth of the vagina and uterus and the beginning of menstruation are delayed.

There is no 'normal'—the range is wide —but because our culture stresses youth and physical appearance the boy or girl who is a late maturer is penalized. Late maturers may need support from caring adults such as parents and teachers and the reassurance that they will sooner or later mature to be like their friends, for they often feel awkward and unattractive to others.

# Menstruation

Menstruation is a monthly discharge from the womb (uterus). In our society we tend to perceive the time that a girl has her first menstrual period as an indication that she has reached puberty. In many societies a girl's first menstruation is an occasion for celebrations, as it indicates that she has now become a woman. From this time on she is thought to be capable of bearing children.

This belief isn't quite correct: the first months of menstruation are usually but not always 'anovulatory', which means that no ovum (egg) is released from the ovary, although the hormones which control ovulation are being formed. Then, quite quickly, the menstrual cycles become ovulatory, and the girl can become pregnant.

Menstrual bleeding occurs because the lining (called the endometrium) of the uterus breaks up and is expelled, together with a small amount of blood and fluid which has oozed from the endometrium into the vagina. It is the end of a complex series of interlocked events which have been preparing the uterus for a possible pregnancy. If the pregnancy fails to occur, the prepared lining is shed and the cycle starts all over again. This is called the menstrual cycle, and it is a process which continues from about the age of thirteen, when the periods start, until about the age of fifty, when they finish. Although the average age for starting menstruation is thirteen, it is normal for it to begin at any age between nine and sixteen. The time of the first menstruation is called the *menarche*.

Usually, menstruation occurs every twenty-eight or twenty-nine days and the bleeding lasts for about four or five days, but shorter or longer intervals can occur and still be normal. It is considered normal for a woman's period to occur at intervals of twenty-two to forty days. This interval is calculated by counting from the first day of bleeding of one menstrual cycle to the first day of bleeding of the next cycle. A period is also considered to be normal if the bleeding only lasts for one day instead of the usual four.

As the **hypothalamus** (the part of the brain which controls the menstrual cycle) is itself influenced by other factors, such as mental stress, emotional upsets, ill health or travel, occasionally it may not send out the messages in the right sequence. If this happens, menstruation may start early or

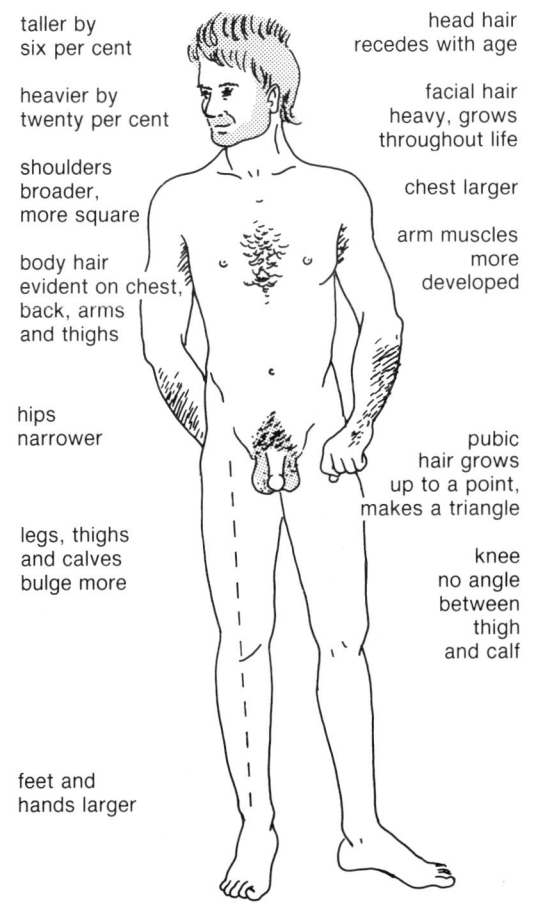

taller by six per cent

heavier by twenty per cent

shoulders broader, more square

body hair evident on chest, back, arms and thighs

hips narrower

legs, thighs and calves bulge more

feet and hands larger

head hair recedes with age

facial hair heavy, grows throughout life

chest larger

arm muscles more developed

pubic hair grows up to a point, makes a triangle

knee no angle between thigh and calf

Sexual characteristics of a young man in his early twenties

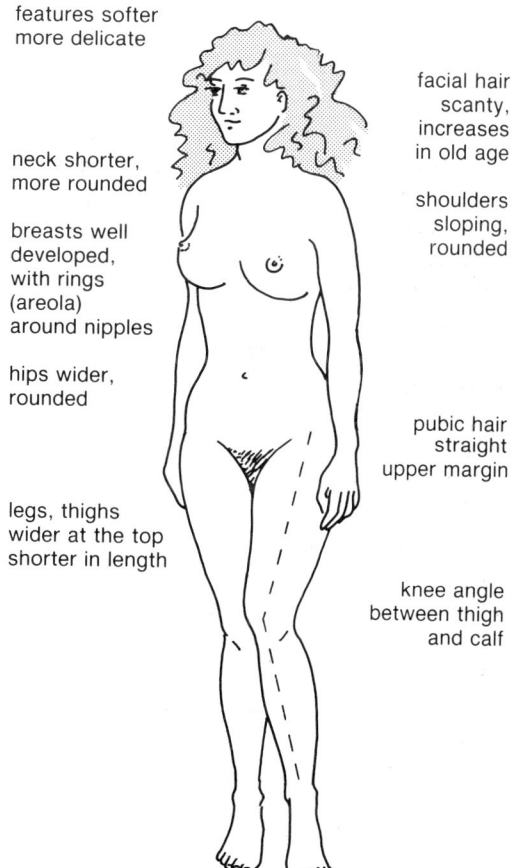

features softer more delicate

neck shorter, more rounded

breasts well developed, with rings (areola) around nipples

hips wider, rounded

legs, thighs wider at the top shorter in length

facial hair scanty, increases in old age

shoulders sloping, rounded

pubic hair straight upper margin

knee angle between thigh and calf

Sexual characteristics of a young woman in her early twenties

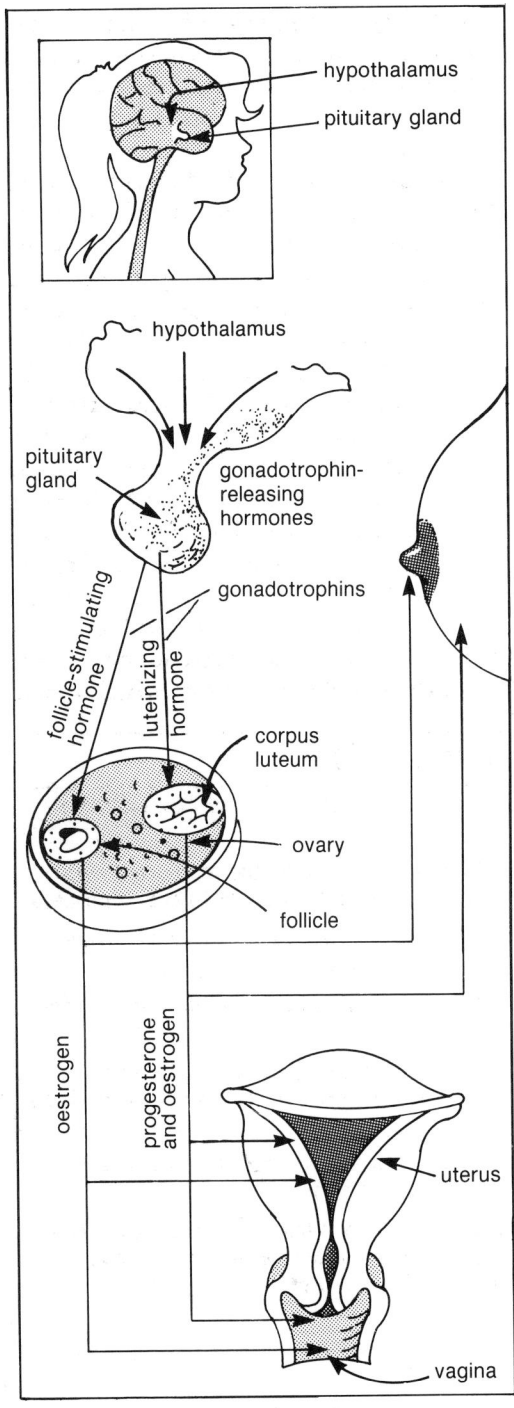

hypothalamus

pituitary gland

hypothalamus

pituitary gland

gonadotrophin-releasing hormones

gonadotrophins

follicle-stimulating hormone

luteinizing hormone

corpus luteum

ovary

follicle

oestrogen

progesterone and oestrogen

uterus

vagina

The control of menstruation

be delayed. So if you become ill, are very upset or very excited, or if you travel, you may have an unusually early or late menstrual period.

Over sixty per cent of young women feel abdominal discomfort, 'heaviness', or crampy pains either just before or during the first one or two days of menstruation. The medical name for menstrual cramps is dysmenorrhoea. Dysmenorrhoea may occur each time the woman menstruates or only sometimes. In fifteen per cent of young women the cramps are so severe that the woman feels ill. The cramps are due to the release by the uterus of a substance called prostaglandin, which makes the uterus contract. This causes the pain. Mild cramps are usually relieved by aspirin, but severe cramps need stronger medicine. Two kinds are available. The Pill is the first, and it usually relieves the dysmenorrhoea but has to be taken every day for most of the menstrual cycle. The second drug is called an anti-prostaglandin; it needs to be taken only when the cramps start.

# The menstrual cycle

The ultimate controller of the menstrual cycle is an area of the brain called the hypothalamus. It sends messages to the pituitary gland with the result that hormones, the gonadotrophins, are released. You may remember that the ovaries contain about 400 000 'primitive' egg cells. Given the right stimulus, any of these cells can grow. Gonadotrophins make this happen.

Each month, after puberty, until the periods cease at the menopause, about twenty of the cells start growing. As they grow they produce oestrogen in increasing amounts and this gets into the bloodstream.

Oestrogen has several important functions. It makes a girl's breasts grow so that they become full and rounded, with well-developed nipples. It makes the lining of the uterus grow, in readiness for possible pregnancy. It helps to keep a woman's vagina moist and clean. It 'feeds back' to the hypothalamus, regulating the release of gonadotrophin.

The amount of oestrogen produced increases as the egg cells grow. These egg cells are now called **follicles**. About twelve days after the day the last menstrual period started, the follicles produce a sudden flood, or surge, of oestrogen. Much of this surge is produced by the one follicle which has grown more quickly and has become much bigger than the others.

The surge of oestrogen enters the blood and 'feeds back' to the hypothalamus. This causes the hypothalamus to send a message to the pituitary gland to release a second gonadotrophin hormone.

This hormone, called progesterone, acts on the biggest egg cell, which has reached the surface of the ovary by now, and the egg or ovum bursts out. The woman has ovulated. It is now about fourteen days from the first day of her last period.

If a woman makes love during the two or three days around the time of ovulation and neither she nor the man uses contraceptives, a pregnancy is likely to occur. For this reason it may be important to know when ovulation occurs in menstrual cycles which are of various lengths. As we discussed earlier, a woman's menstrual cycle is rarely exactly twenty-eight days long. It is 'normal' for a woman to have a menstrual period at an interval which varies from twenty-two to forty days. Because of this variation, ovulation occurs at different times in different cycles. The most constant way of calculating when ovulation has occurred is to count back fourteen days from the first day of the menstrual period.

## Facts about menstruation

- Periods usually start between the ages of twelve and fifteen, but a year or two earlier or later is normal.

- For the first year or two, the periods may occur irregularly, but soon the menstrual cycle becomes regular and menstruation normally occurs every twenty-eight or twenty-nine days.

- A girl can use a vaginal tampon or a sanitary pad, to protect her clothes from menstrual discharge. She can choose which suits her circumstances. Both are equally safe.

- Some people experience feelings of tension, depression, restlessness and tiredness in the two or three days before menstruation.

- Most women can usually do anything during menstruation they do when they are not menstruating, provided they feel comfortable. This includes sport, entertainment and, if the woman chooses, sex.

- Emotions can affect menstruation, as can changes in routine. The changes may stop menstruation, make the periods irregular or produce heavier periods.

- Some women have painful, crampy periods. These occur only if the woman has ovulated. Often aspirin helps, but if the pain is severe and persistent the woman should consult a doctor who will prescribe anti-prostaglandin drugs which usually relieve the pain.

When should you visit a doctor?
- If you miss two or more periods

- If you start bleeding, or spotting between periods

- If your periods are very heavy, often with clots

- If your periods last for more than eight days.

Even then ovulation may occur one or two days before that day or two days after it. Some women know when they ovulate as they experience a pain in the abdomen which lasts a few hours. Other women find that the character of their vaginal secretions changes: the amount increases and it becomes clear and stretchable when a woman puts some between her first finger and thumb and then separates them. Knowledge of the changes in vaginal secretions which occur at the time of ovulation is necessary if a woman decides to use the mucus method for contraception. (See p. 60.)

The follicle from which the ovum has escaped collapses and turns yellow. Its cells now produce a second sex hormone, progesterone, as well as oestrogen. Progesterone increases the succulence of the endometrium, so that it is more ready to receive the fertilized egg if pregnancy should occur. It also acts on the breasts, so that they become bigger for a few days before menstruation. (Some women have quite painful breasts in the week before menstruation.)

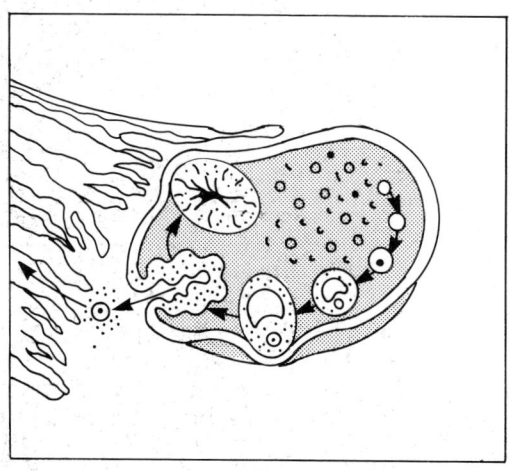

The growth of a follicle during the menstrual cycle

Unless pregnancy occurs, the collapsed follicle ceases producing hormones. The amount of oestrogen and progesterone in the blood falls, and the endometrium crumbles. A menstrual period starts.

Then the whole process begins again.

# Menstruation

In some societies a menstruating woman is kept separate from the rest of the group. This is because the people believe that her menstrual blood will pollute the food, or the ground. In our society women are not segregated when they are menstruating but most people still find it difficult to discuss menstruation. Menstruation is seen as a 'taboo' subject, rather 'dirty', rather 'unhygienic'. This is emphasized by the names given to menstruation: 'the poorly time', 'the curse', 'the rags'.

To absorb the menstrual flow during menstruation, women may choose from the following: a sanitary pad or napkin; a minipad; or a tampon.

Most young women use pads, at least initially, but later may decide to change to tampons. Pads and minipads cover the area around the vaginal entrance and absorb menstrual flow. They are kept in place by an adhesive backing which is attached to the pants. Pads are rather bulky and the young woman often worries that they may show if she wears tight fitting clothes or jeans. If the menstrual flow is light, the woman may choose to wear a minipad. Minipads absorb less flow but may feel more comfortable. The third method is for the woman to insert a tampon into her vagina. Tampons are made of absorbent material in several sizes, and are cylindrical in shape. A string is attached to the tampon for easy removal. Tampons should be changed about every 4 to 6

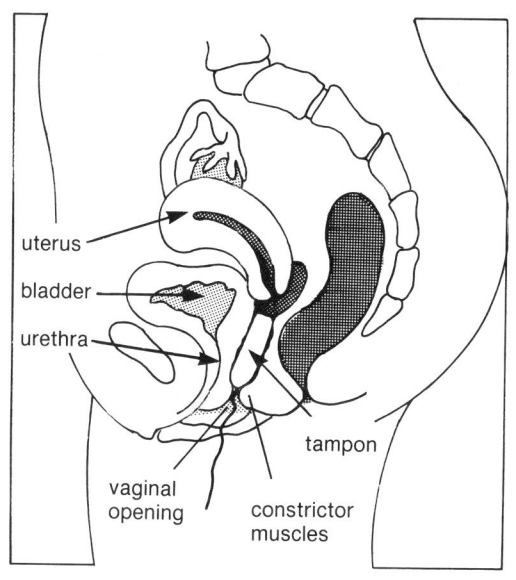

uterus

bladder

urethra

tampon

vaginal opening

constrictor muscles

The position of a tampon in the vagina

hours. They can be used by virgins, as in most cases the tampon does not damage the hymen. Some young women can insert a tampon easily; others need a little practice before they become used to doing it. The tampon should be inserted up the vagina beyond the muscles around the entrance so that it can't be felt when it is in place.

A woman often chooses a tampon because it is more practical. First, she feels she can wear whatever clothes she likes, including a bikini or a leotard. The tampon won't be seen. Second, she can go swimming with freedom, knowing that the tampon will absorb all the menstrual flow. Third, there is no menstrual odour, as the menstrual

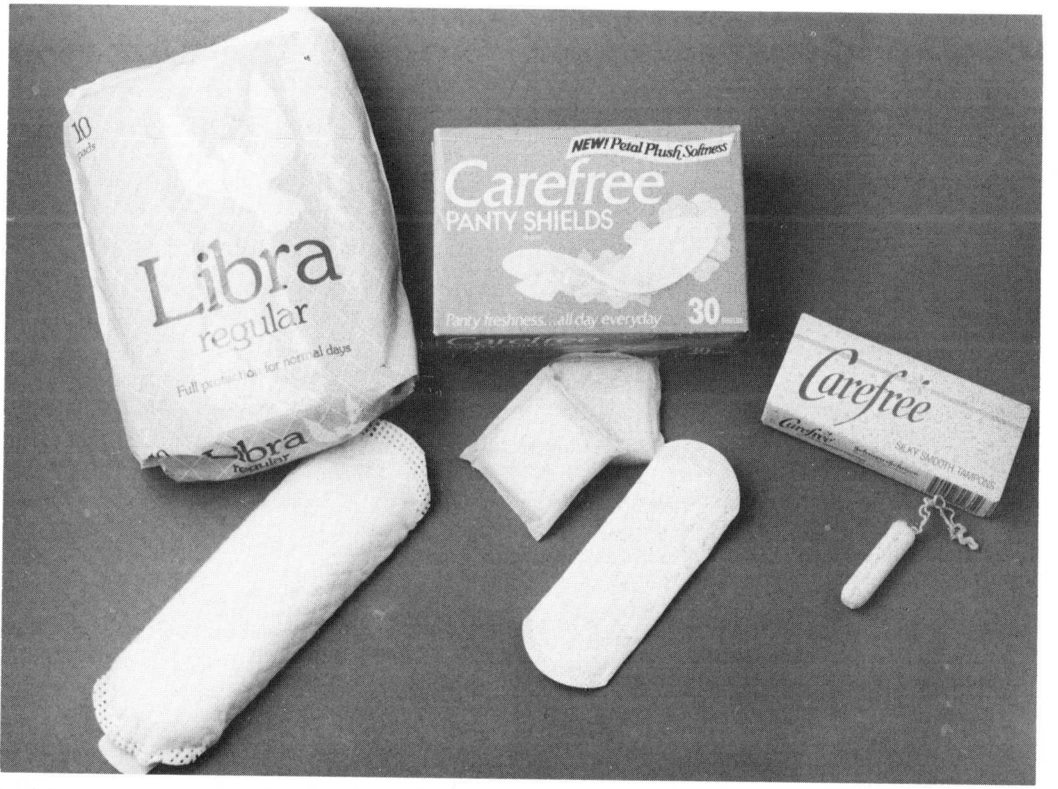

A sanitary pad, a minipad and a tampon (left to right)

flow is absorbed inside the body. Fourth, a day's supply of tampons easily fits in a purse or handbag.

Some women worry about using tampons. They are afraid the tampon will fall out. It won't, because it is held in place by the muscles of the pelvis. They are afraid it may 'get lost inside'. It won't, because the vagina ends at the cervix and the string enables a woman to pull the tampon out. They are afraid that tampons may cause the toxic shock syndrome or TSS. It is true that a few cases of TSS have been reported following tampon use. If a woman washes her hands before inserting the tampon, and changes it every four hours, unwrapping the new, clean tampon just before using it, TSS is unlikely to occur. TSS has received a great deal of publicity but is a very rare occurrence. Although most reports have related tampon use to TSS, the illness may occur from other causes. In certain conditions a germ called golden staph (*Staphylococcus aureus*) releases a toxin which is absorbed into the person's blood. If this happens, the person feels ill, develops a high fever, vomiting, muscle pains, and a sunburn-like red rash over all the body. The rash fades, but about two weeks later the skin on the palms of the hands begins to peel. In some people the blood pressure falls, they become shocked, and can die.

# Adolescence and development

In spite of popular belief, adolescence is not a time when one rejects all one's parents' values and beliefs. It is a time when an individual, swept by hormonal tides, conscious of a new-found sexuality, is trying to answer the question 'Who am I?' It is a time when, quite properly, the young person begins to question, and to argue. It is the time when a boy or a girl begins to formulate his or her own beliefs and values and wants to have the chance to make decisions, to choose; it is a time when young people want to test out their fantasies and to begin to make their own realities. It is a time of transition, of great inward and outward change.

Adjustment to change is often difficult. It becomes easier when the adolescent is secure and is part of a family which encourages discussion and which understands that he or she is uncertain about how to behave. Adjustment is more difficult if the teenager's parents demand conformity, always 'knows best', oppose any attempt the teenager makes to express personal views, and attempt to dominate him or her. Adjustment is still more difficult if the parents ignore the teenager's behaviour, or offer only minimal guidance, so that the teenager is unsure whether what he or she is doing has their approval.

Adjustment is certainly easiest if the teenagers and their parents can discuss matters which seem important openly and easily, in friendship and love. Discussing means listening! Many people hear but don't listen; unless a person listens he or she will never understand. That applies to teenagers and to their parents!

Discussion between young people and their parents has to include sexuality, because there may be differences in the attitudes of parents and teenagers to sexuality. Many teenagers today question the belief that young people should not have sex before marriage and should be faithful to their partner after marriage. They see some of their contemporaries enjoying sexual relationships, they read of the number of divorces in society, and observe the anger and tensions between some of the adults they meet.

Most teenagers also reject the concept that sex is just an appetite to be satisfied as the opportunity arises, with any available partner and without any emotional involvement. Older people tend to believe that this is how most teenagers behave. They are wrong. A few teenagers are sexual adventurers, enjoying one-night stands without any emotional involvement. Some adults also are sexual adventurers.

Most teenagers approach sexuality with concern. They want to be close to, to touch and to enjoy their loved one, even if the love may fade after a longer or a shorter time. The experience is a learning experience in which the two teenagers are developing their personalities. They may both want and enjoy sexual intercourse, but it is sex with an emotional involvement, with a loved one, not sex as an appetite, to be gratified and forgotten—until the next time.

Beliefs about sexual behaviour vary very much from family to family and depend very much on the society in which you live. In China, for example, most men and women remain chaste until they marry, and that rarely occurs before the woman is aged twenty-four. In India childhood marriages are still arranged, but the couple do not live together until the girl is sixteen or thereabouts. In some Mediterranean countries girls are expected to remain virgins until marriage and it is a disgrace for the family if an unmarried girl has sex but young men are not expected to be chaste and, in the towns at least, may have sex, often with prostitutes. Of course these attitudes towards sex vary within countries and from person to person. Each person has his or her own particular beliefs and you may encounter many attitudes different from your own. You should respect these beliefs.

# Adolescence and sexual behaviour

How do adolescents behave sexually? Most people accept that young people 'neck' and that many enjoy 'heavy petting'. Many parents are very concerned that their children, particularly their daughters, 'have gone all the way' and have had sexual intercourse.

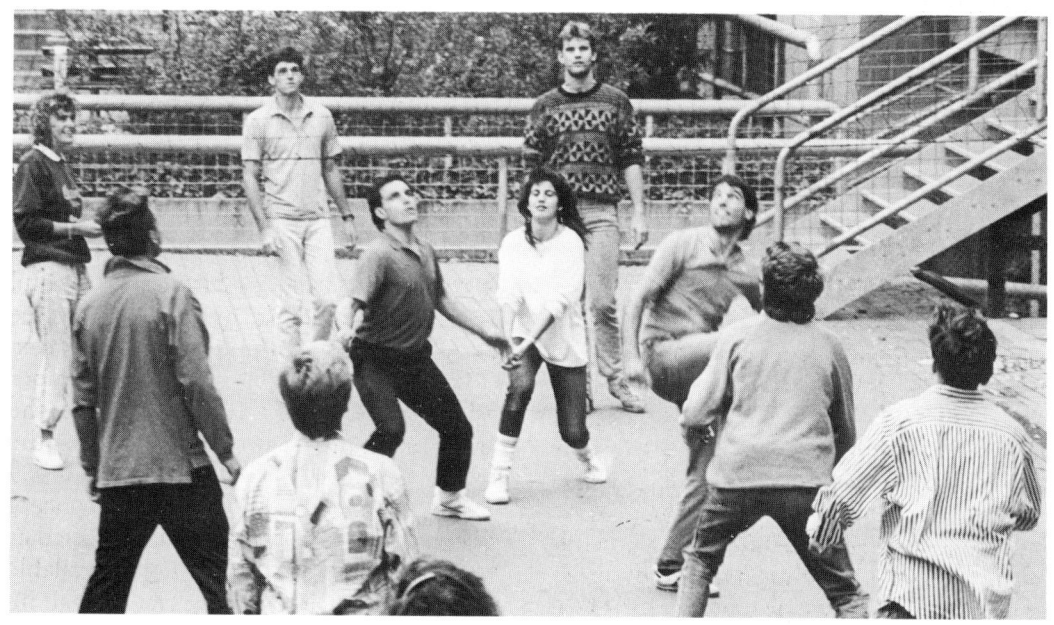

Are today's young people more sexually permissive than two or three generations ago? Or do they just talk about sex more?

It is difficult to find the answer. As sexual expression is so personal most people keep their sexual behaviour to themselves, and don't talk about it. In the past, young men were expected (sometimes encouraged) to have sexual experiences, whilst young women were expected to remain virgins until marriage. This implies that the young men must have paid prostitutes for sex (and often acquired a sexually transmitted disease for free); or had sex with married women (which made them adulterers); or have used a girl acquaintance who was known to be an 'easy lay'.

This was, and is, the double standard of sexual behaviour. It is based on the false belief that men need sex more than women; that they have to have sex to relieve sexual tensions; and that the experience helps them 'educate' their virgin bride when they marry.

In 1966 an American professor of sociology, Dr Reiss divided young people's sexual behaviour into four groups, depending on their attitudes to sexuality.

The groups are:

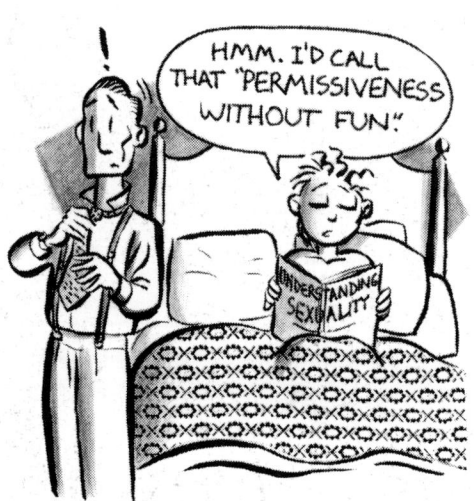

## Abstinence

Kissing and some petting are allowed but premarital sexual intercourse is forbidden for both sexes.

## The double standard

Men, having a stronger sexual drive than women, may 'indulge' in sexual intercourse when they want. Women should wait for marriage, or occasionally may have sexual intercourse with a fiance, because of his urgent needs.

## Permissiveness with affection

The couple have an affectionate, relatively stable relationship, and believe there is nothing morally wrong in having and enjoying sexual intercourse.

## Permissiveness without affection

Sex is fun and gives pleasure, to both men and women. Each can enjoy sexual intercourse regardless of the amount of affection that exists between the partners.

The proportion of teenagers who behave in one or other of these ways is not easy to determine. No reliable surveys of adolescent sexual behaviour have been made in Australia, but several have been carried out in Britain, Scandinavia and the USA in the last ten years. These indicate that about one-third of teenaged men and women avoid sexual intercourse until they are married, although they may enjoy heavy petting. One in every five teenaged men and women still accepts the double standard of sexual behaviour. About one-third of teenagers have relationships during which they have sexual intercourse. The relationship may end and the couples

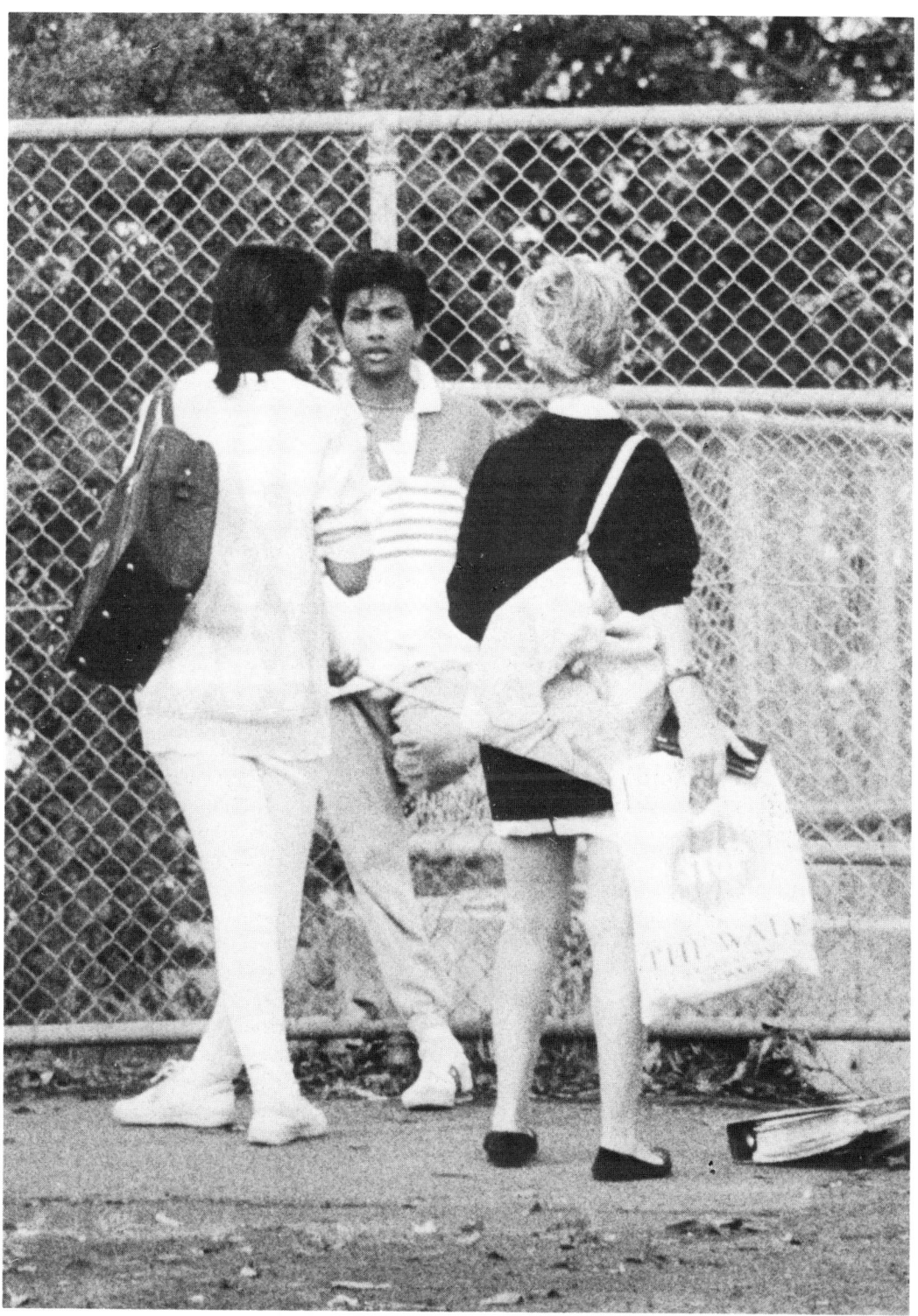

may find other partners with whom they have a relationship which includes sexual intercourse, but during each relationship they remain faithful to their partner. Finally, about one in seven teenagers are sexual adventurers, enjoying sexual intercourse with several partners, regardless of the amount of affection between them. In the past more teenaged males than females behaved sexually in this way, but today the proportions are about the same.

In the past twenty years an increasing number of teenaged men and women began to have sexual intercourse, either within a relationship which lasts for months or years, or as sexual adventurers. Over this period, more teenaged women began to have sex at an earlier age. In spite of these findings, there is no suggestion that most teenagers are sexually permissive. Most teenage relationships are conducted with dignity and with concern for the other person.

# Consequences of adolescent sexual relationships

What is disturbing from the surveys into adolescent sexual behaviour is that a large number of teenagers do not know the time during a woman's menstrual cycle when pregnancy is most likely to occur, and a large number do not use contraceptives. This means that unexpected, unwanted pregnancies occur.

In 1983 over one million American teenagers, or about one adolescent girl in every ten, became pregnant. Of this number 600 000 gave birth, and half of them (25 per cent of all pregnant teenagers) were unmarried at the time of birth. Alone, they had to cope with the problems of early child-rearing. Over 450 000 teenagers, 43 per

cent of all who became pregnant, had an abortion to terminate an unwanted pregnancy. In Britain in 1983 the numbers of premarital pregnancies were fewer, partly because the population is smaller, but only 31 per cent were followed by marriage. In 27 per cent the mother remained single and in nearly 37 per cent the pregnancy was terminated by an abortion. In Australia, in 1983, 29 500 teenaged women, or one in every 21, became pregnant. About 21 per cent gave birth after marrying (although half married after becoming pregnant). Thirty-five per cent gave birth but didn't marry. Five per cent had a miscarriage, and 39 per cent—over 11 000 young women—had the pregnancy aborted.

Several problems arise from teenaged pregnancy. It is known that teenaged marriages are particularly unstable, four in every ten breaking down within seven years, at a time when children are particularly vulnerable to psychological disturbances. Although a single mother is less discriminated against today than she was ten years ago, she has a more difficult life and has a greater chance of being depressed. The presence of a young child means she may be unable to acquire additional education or skills to help improve her life style. Abortion performed in the first ten weeks of pregnancy, in a clinic or hospital, is a safe procedure, and although most women consider carefully before having an abortion, guilt often follows.

These reasons add force to the belief that sexually active teenagers should obtain contraceptive advice and use contraceptives before they start having sex.

In the countries mentioned earlier, over two-thirds of the pregnancies and half the births were not intended.

Two solutions to the problem of unwanted pregnancy are possible. The first is for young people to change their sexual behaviour so that neither young men nor young women have sex before marriage. This is unlikely to occur.

The second is to be sure that teenagers understand their sexuality and behave responsibly sexually. Sexual responsibility means that neither partner is exploited or treated as a sex object by the other; it also means that sexual intercourse does not take place unless one or other of the couple is using a reliable contraceptive.

# Choices in sexual behaviour

How you behave sexually is something you will have to decide for yourself.

If your choice is that you do not wish to have sexual intercourse before you marry, you have the right to expect that your choice will be respected by your friends, and that you will not be pressured into having sexual intercourse.

You may choose to have a sexual relationship with a person for whom you have real affection. During the relationship it is likely that neither of you will have any other sexual partner. As you are in love probably you will both want to be sure that an unwanted pregnancy is avoided. You can be sure of this if one or other of you uses a reliable contraceptive when you both decide you want to have sexual intercourse.

Some teenagers alternate between several partners, having sex with them in a random way. They are not in love with the partners, but enjoy sex for its pleasurable sensations. These relationships may lead to an unwanted pregnancy or to the acquisition of a sexually transmitted disease. In both instances the consequences can be grave. People who are sexual adventurers should be responsible enough to make sure

that they or their partners are using contraceptives. The chance of acquiring a sexually transmitted disease increases with the number of sexual partners, as one or other may have an infection and be unaware of it, or worse, may be infected and know about it, but persist in having sexual intercourse (or oral sex). A person who has a sexually transmitted disease and has not been treated and cured is likely to give that disease to his or her sexual partner if they have sexual intercourse. This action is sexually irresponsible.

*Investigations*
● Find out some of the beliefs (past and present, in this culture and in others) associated with menstruation. Do you know, or can you suggest, the origins of these beliefs?

*Discussions*
● What are some of the common names for menstruation?
● On a piece of paper, write down anonymously those things about your own sexuality which make you feel good, and on another piece of paper those things which make you feel bad. Have a team leader or teacher compile a composite list and discuss.

*Activities*
● Put a tampon in a glass of water and see it change size.
● Observe and record evidence of the variations in human development during adolescence. You can do this by recording the heights and weights of class members of the same age.

# 4

# SEXUAL AWAKENING AND AROUSAL

With puberty and adolescence a person's sexuality becomes much more intense. He or she becomes sexually awakened, and becomes sexually aroused much more readily and easily. The arousal may occur during sleep, when a man may have a 'wet dream', or it may be felt as a need to masturbate, particularly in response to the stimulus of erotic thoughts and fantasies, of looking at erotic pictures, or of reading erotic literature.

## Sexual arousal

What is it that makes one person want to talk to, to touch, and to be with another special person? We don't know, but there is a theory that seems to fit the facts. This theory was first developed by Dr Stoller, a Californian psychiatrist.

Dr Stoller believes that each person makes up his or her own 'sexual arousal script', rather like a television writer makes up a television script. Each of us is the hero or the heroine of our own script. The story is based on childhood experiences, on memories and on fantasies. As the person grows and has more experiences, the 'script' is continually rewritten, some parts are omitted, others expanded, until each person has created his or her unique script. This script identifies the type of individual who excites the 'writer' sexually.

If a person meets the type of individual he or she has created in the script, sexual arousal may occur. If the other person has created a similar arousal script, then he or she responds. The response may be by words, but usually is by a gesture or some other form of body language.

The couple meet and explore each other's personality and character. They either become closer, which means they want to see more of each other and perhaps they fall in love, or else the excitement fades and they separate, seeking another person who fits their script better.

In the sexual arousal script all the five senses are involved, but, in our culture, sight seems to be the most important sense, especially for males. A male is turned on, to start with, more by the appearance of a female than by the sound of her voice, the smell of her body, the taste of her lips or by her touch. (It used to be believed that women were more sexually aroused by a man's character than by his looks. It is now known that this isn't true.)

But even if the person looks attractive, an ugly voice or sweaty smell may, on closer acquaintance, reduce the sexual arousal. Body touch, on the other hand, usually increases the initial sexual arousal.

The body has zones which are particularly sexually arousing (erotic). In our culture the breasts, the buttocks and the genitals are the most stimulating erotic zones (facts which have not remained unnoticed by advertisers).

# Myths about masturbation

| Myth | Fact |
|---|---|
| • Masturbation is an abnormal way of behaving; it is evil. | • If it is abnormal, nearly 100 per cent of boys and 75 per cent of girls are abnormal because they masturbate. |
| • Masturbation is unhealthy and is evidence of emotional immaturity. | • Masturbation is normal and healthy. Most people masturbate at some time or other throughout their lives. They are not emotionally immature. |
| • You can damage your health by masturbating too much. | • Masturbation has never done physical harm to anyone. |
| • People who masturbate will develop sexual problems when they marry. | • The truth is the opposite. People who don't masturbate are more likely to have sexual problems when they marry. |
| • Masturbation is unnatural, it is self-abuse. | • Rubbish. Many people want to be alone, to experience the sensations of music, nature or poetry—or sexual stimulation. |
| • Masturbation stunts your growth, weakens your brain, makes you blind, brings on disease. | • This rubbish was propagated particularly by numbers of sour medical men in Queen Victoria's reign, and it as much rubbish now as it was then. |

Masturbation is a normal, healthy sexual outlet.

Other areas of the body are erotic for some people. Some people become sexually aroused by having their hair stroked or brushed; others by having their necks or ears nibbled; others by having their backs, feet or arms massaged.

By mid-adolescence a person's sexual arousal script is nearly complete; from now on it is less likely to be rewritten. By this time each person knows (if only subconsciously) the kind of person that he or she finds sexually arousing, and will look for and try to make contact with such a person.

## Wet dreams

One of the earliest signs that sexual arousal has begun to increase is that boys and girls begin to have sexual dreams. The dreams are confused fantasies and, in the case of boys, may end with a sudden ejaculation, a 'wet dream'.

Wet dreams are normal. They show that sexual awakening has begun. As alternative sexual outlets become possible, such as masturbation or sexual intercourse, wet dreams occur less frequently, but they may recur at any time of life.

## Masturbation

A common way in which a person finds pleasure from sexual arousal fantasies is by fondling, caressing or stroking his or her own genitals. This is masturbation. By the age of fifteen most boys have masturbated and many masturbate frequently. Fewer girls masturbate, perhaps because the clitoris is less obviously accessible than the penis.

Masturbation is a normal sexual outlet and an important sexual learning process. It is a preparation for adult sexuality. The boy or girl learns the shape and feel of his or her own sexual organs. They learn their smell and the pleasurable physical sensations obtained by caressing them. During masturbation, a person builds up a fantasy world and exercises the imagination in an erotic (sexual) manner. Masturbation used to be called 'self-abuse' or 'the solitary vice', but there is no truth that it is harmful in any way. In spite of this scientific knowledge, many parents condemn or punish their children if they find them masturbating and make them feel undeservedly guilty about their behaviour, and myths persist about the dangers of masturbation.

# Petting

Petting is an American word which implies that the couple enjoy love play which includes everything except sexual intercourse. Light petting (or necking) is love play in which anything above the waist may be touched, but the clothed parts of the body are only touched through the clothes. In heavy petting the unclothed body is touched, kissed or caressed, and the genital area may be fondled. Either or both partners may have an orgasm, helped by the other, but they don't have sexual intercourse.

Petting is also enjoyed by couples who may follow it by sexual intercourse, when it is referred to as 'foreplay'. I believe that

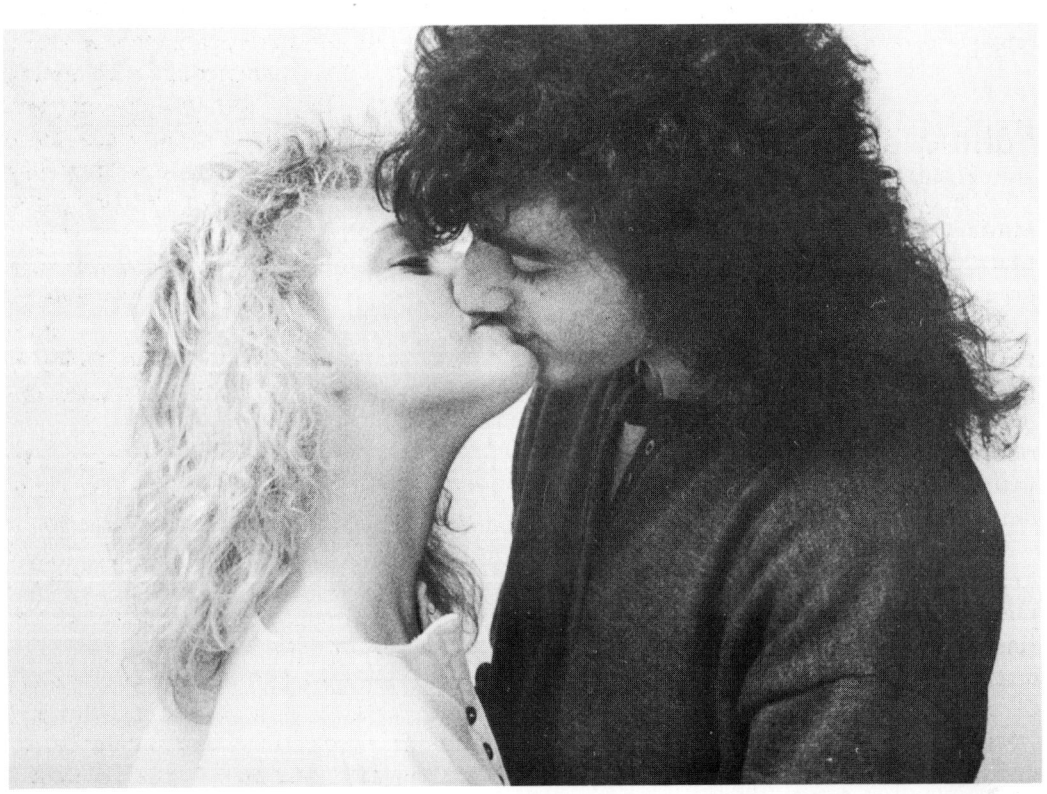

this word should be avoided as it implies that all love play must inevitably lead to sexual intercourse (otherwise what is foreplay before?). It needn't. Couples may be content to pet heavily. A phrase which communicates the idea better is 'mutual pleasuring'.

Petting (and mutual pleasuring) give people the opportunity to explore each other's bodies, including the sexual organs, and to interact emotionally with each other. It helps the partners discover each other's erotic body areas and to talk to each other. It helps each of the couple to be more sensitive and receptive to the other's sexual desires and needs.

Most adolescents enjoy petting, which may be light or heavy. In the United States, studies by Dr Kinsey show that twenty-five years ago over one-third of boys and one-quarter of girls petted heavily and had orgasms from the experience. Today more than half of all young men and women engage in petting.

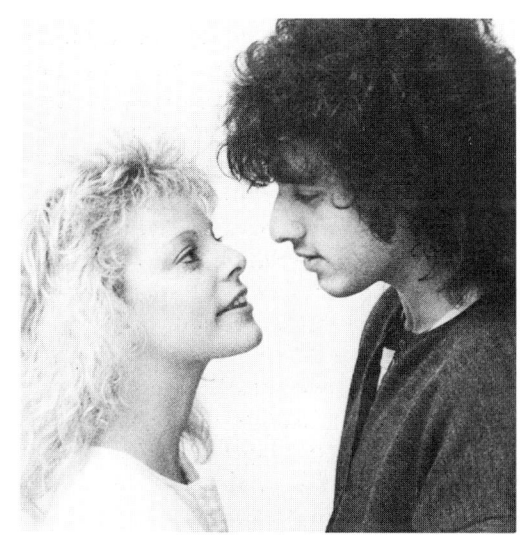

# Falling in love

Love is not easy to define. The poet Rainer Maria Rilke wrote: 'Love consists of this—that two solitudes protect and touch and greet each other.'

Love is the very personal emotion in sexual arousal. It transcends the need for a physical relief of sexual tension, adding to it a desire to please and to protect the loved one. Love unites an urgent sexual drive with a deep emotional passion and a tender respect and caring for the loved one.

You have to learn to express your love. Learning to express love begins in early puberty, with fantasies of love and marriage with a popular 'hero'. Later there are crushes and crazes (often for older people) of the opposite or same sex. Then come intense friendships between people of similar ages, when both believe they are in love,

but are, in fact, not ready or able to make a permanent commitment to each other. For a time they are inseparable. They do the same things, they want to be together, they long for one another's presence when they are apart. They spend hours telephoning each other. They enjoy long petting sessions, learning to share their sexual emotional and physical experiences. They may have sexual intercourse or they may not. After a time the passion passes, the friendship fades, the love seems lost and they part, perhaps painfully. This relationship may be succeeded by another intense friendship, and another period of 'being in love'. These special friendships wax and wane as time passes.

All these experiences help teenagers to obtain greater insight into their own emotional and physical needs, and to match this up with the needs of another. The experiences help young people to learn what they most value in themselves and in the 'important other'.

These experiences usually enable deeper, longer-lasting friendships to arise, which in turn may develop into an overwhelming affection for a particular

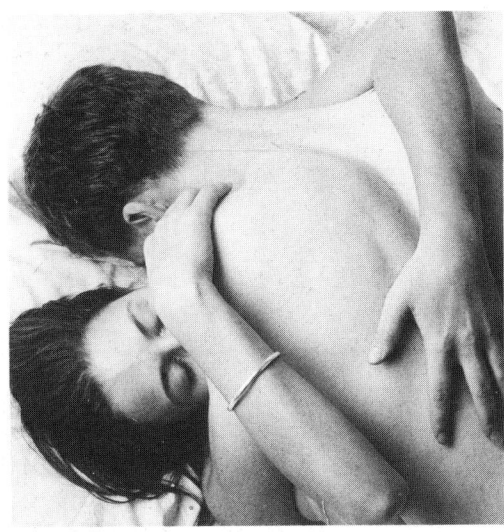

'other', which grows in strength until both people believe they are in love. If each partner's awareness of the other is based on reality, not on a fantasy of what the other *ought* to be, the love most probably will last.

# Sexual intercourse

Most parents now accept that their children probably will masturbate and are likely to pet, but are very concerned if their adolescent children have sexual intercourse. They may believe that sex before marriage is morally wrong; if they have a daughter they may fear that she might be exploited or become pregnant; and they may fear that their daughter or their son may contract a sexually transmitted disease.

Studies in the USA, Scandinavia and Britain have shown that premarital sexual intercourse is increasingly common amongst teenagers. With this knowledge, many parents are coming to accept that their children will have sexual intercourse

and to encourage their son or daughter to talk with them beforehand, so that they can discuss together the possible consequences of premarital sex.

The different attitudes to sexual intercourse held by a teenager's parents and by his or her friends can cause conflicts, which can lead to emotional insecurity. The pressures by young men on young women to permit sexual intercourse can be intense and difficult for the young woman to handle, as she may feel that she will 'lose' the man if she refuses. The decision whether to have sexual intercourse or to remain a virgin is hers alone. It is unwise for anyone to enter into a sexual relationship just because their friends are doing it, or because the man is putting on the pressure. You are ready for a complete sexual relationship when you have decided that you are comfortable and secure, not when you feel that you must do as your friends do or run the risk of being rejected and scorned by them.

Sexual intercourse is usually thought of as the pinnacle of human sexuality, and for most people it is. But it should be seen for what it is: the culmination of a sequence of sexually stimulating events during which both partners receive and give pleasure to the other and express their loving feelings. To many young men the objective is a quick get it in, get it out, and go home. If both partners get sexual pleasure from this no emotional problem arises. But, if that is all sex consists of, many women feel that they are being used, and are being treated as objects, not as people. A young woman has the right to refuse a demand for sexual intercourse. She has the right to say 'No!', and should say no, if she does not feel ready for sexual intercourse. 'No' is a very good oral contraceptive. If human sexuality is perceived as merely exploiting a partner for one's own selfish pleasure, without trying to return that pleasure, the humanity of sexuality is destroyed. It becomes a mechanical insensitive exploitation of another person.

Sexual intercourse is not a competitive indoor sport to be boasted about later (usually embroidered with lies), but a warm pleasurable experience between two turned-on people.

As we have seen earlier, sexual intercourse should not be attempted until the woman's vagina is well lubricated and the 'sex cushions' have formed. To attempt sexual intercourse before lubrication has occurred, particularly if it is the first time a girl has had sexual intercourse, is insensitive, as it may be painful for her. This can be avoided if the man is sufficiently aware of a woman's sexual arousal responses, and sensitive enough to appreciate her needs. A sensitive lover will find out what his or her partner finds most stimulating sexually if the couple talk to each other about their feelings and about what each finds **most** enjoyable.

## Sexual positions

No book about human sexuality can ignore the different sexual positions. Starting over 2000 years ago with the *Kama Sutra*, hundreds of books have been written to explain the technique of love-making and to discuss the advantages and disadvantages of the various positions. In spite of apparently infinite variations the sexual

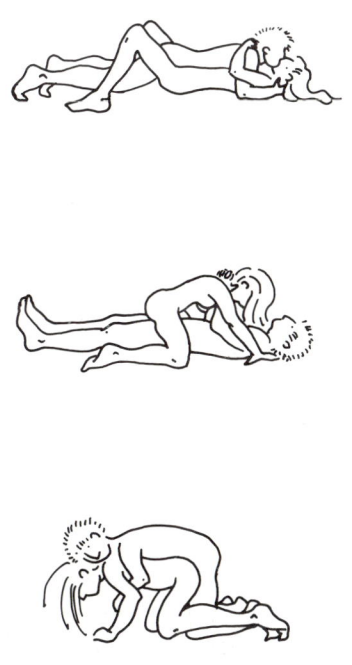

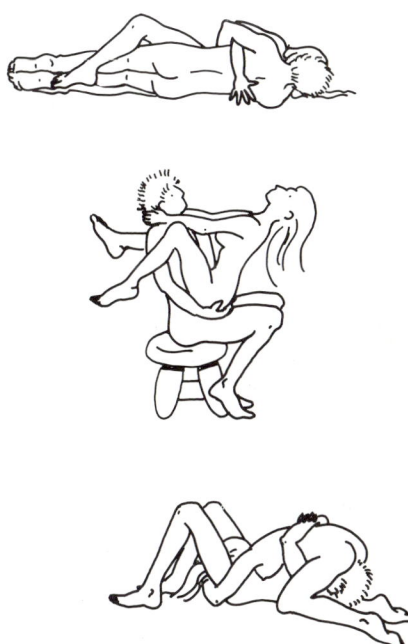

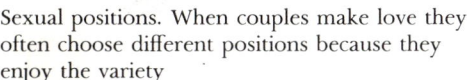

Sexual positions. When couples make love they often choose different positions because they enjoy the variety

39

positions in reality fall into about six groups. These are: **First**, face to face, man on top, the so-called missionary position (because the missionary was on top, the native girl beneath). **Second**, face to face, woman on top. **Third**, the man facing the woman's back, the rear entry position. **Fourth**, face to face, side by side. **Fifth**, sitting positions. And for completeness, **sixth**, the 69 position in which the man licks the woman's clitoris (**cunnilingus**) whilst she sucks his penis (**fellatio**).

Any position the couple enjoys is normal, provided neither is uncomfortable, embarrassed or hurt. Couples who frequently use different positions for variety say it adds to the enjoyment of their sexuality.

Knowledge about sexual positions and skill in using them to pleasure each partner is an important part, but only a small part, of human sexuality, which is not just a sort of sexual athletic contest.

# Oral sex

Oral sex means what it says. One partner in the couple uses the lips, the tongue, or the mouth to stimulate the other's penis or clitoris. When a woman uses oral sex to stimulate a man she licks, kisses and sucks his penis. The lining of the mouth is very soft and sensitive and the woman can use her tongue as well to give the man added sensual pleasure. This is called **fellatio**.

When a man uses his tongue or his lips to lick a woman's clitoral area, he often helps the woman reach orgasm more quickly than if he stimulates her clitoris directly with his finger, or indirectly during sexual intercourse. This is called **cunnilingus**.

Many homosexuals, both male and female, use oral sex as their preferred way of reaching orgasm.

There is nothing new or indecent about oral sex. It has been known about and practised, but perhaps not written about, for at least 5000 years.

Oral sex is a normal way of expressing an intimate sexual relationship between two aroused people. It is safe and enjoyable.

*Investigations*
● Find for yourself some advertisements where sexuality is emphasized to sell a product. What kind of impact do such advertisements have on one or more of your five senses?

*Discussions*
● Do you agree with the statement on p. 37 'You have to learn to express your love'? How do you think people learn to love?
● What is your opinion of Dr Stoller's sexual arousal script? Try to give reasons for your opinion. Think about your own script—what qualities are you looking for in a partner?
● Discuss any pressures to have sexual intercourse that you have experienced. What are your real feelings about having sexual intercourse?

*Activities*
● Find a compatibility quiz in a magazine. Do the questions emphasize the sorts of things you find important in a partner? Devise your own quiz.
● Conduct a survey of students in your school to find the characteristics they look for in a partner—select the ten most often occurring characteristics and rank them.

# 5

# THE HUMAN SEXUAL RESPONSE

In the past hundred years medical scientists have been exploring how the human body works. We have a vast amount of knowledge today about how your heart is regulated, how your hormones are controlled, how you alter your breathing in stressful situations, how you digest your food and what happens to it in your body. The science of physiology has uncovered much, and there is still much more to be known.

Until about twenty-five years ago medical scientists chose to ignore one of the fundamental aspects of human life, the physiology of the human sexual response. Such investigations were thought indecent, indelicate or unworthy of scientific study.

Then, from 1954 onwards, Dr Masters and Dr Johnson investigated the anatomy and physiology of the human sexual response. They showed that it could be studied like any other human physiological activity.

## What sex is for

Human sexuality enables two people to express the emotional feelings for one another through their bodies, and to enjoy mutual sexual pleasure. It also makes possible the creation of new life and the perpetuation of the human race.

Sexual pleasuring need not necessarily include sexual intercourse for both partners to become close, but, if they want to have children, it usually requires that the man obtain an erection and ejaculate within (or around) the woman's vagina.

Sexual pleasuring is important before the couple have sexual intercourse as it leads to considerable physical changes in the genital organs of each partner. These changes make sexual intercourse more pleasurable. For example, although a woman can have sexual intercourse without being sexually aroused, if the vagina is not well lubricated her pleasure is diminished and intercourse may be painful. Sexual intercourse is virtually impossible if the man has not become sexually aroused, and if his body has not undergone certain physical changes, of which the most important is that his penis becomes erect and firm. A man cannot have sexual intercourse with a limp, floppy penis!

## How men and women respond sexually

The changes which occur in the two sexes in response to being sexually aroused or excited are different, but each complements the other. In both sexes the changes are due to an increase in the amount of blood flowing into the genital organs so that they become 'congested', and to a heightening in the 'tone' of the muscles of the body so that they are more tense. The latter occurs later in the progress of sexual

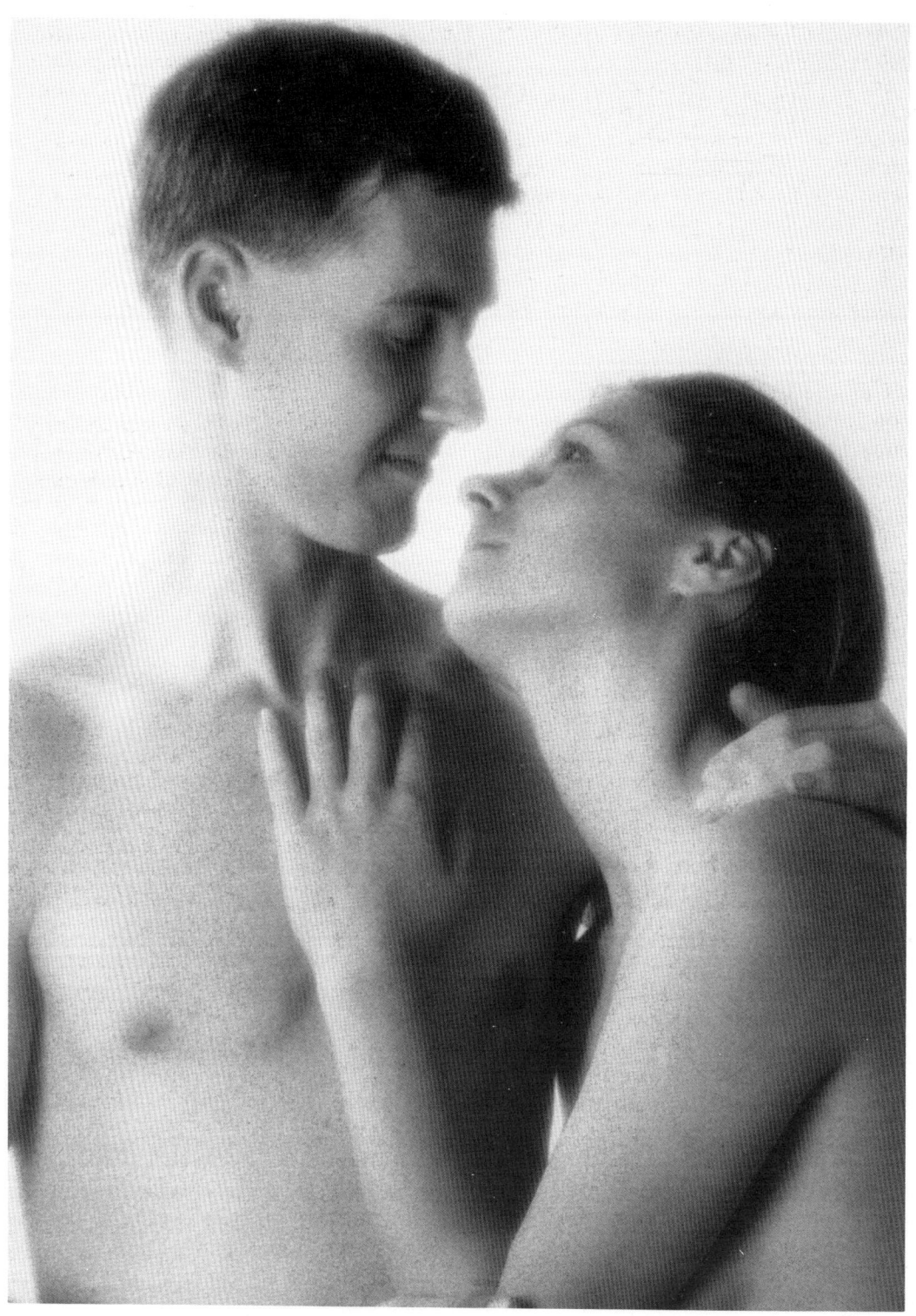

arousal. The blood congestion is the first sign of sexual excitement.

Sexual arousal may occur in several ways. It may occur by thinking about, or seeing, a person to whom you feel attracted. It may occur by looking at erotic pictures or by reading erotic literature. It may occur by masturbating and fantasizing.

A person becomes sexually aroused because messages from a 'sex centre' in the brain pass along the spinal cord to the nerves which control the genital organs.

The message becomes stronger if the erotic parts of the other person's body are fondled. Usually, the erotic parts of the body are the lips, the tongue, a woman's breasts, nipples and genitals, and a man's penis and scrotum, but other parts of the human body may be found to be sexually arousing too. With increasing sexual arousal, sexual excitement occurs, and physical changes occur in the body, making it obvious to each partner that the other is aroused. Each is responding sexually.

# The stages of sexual response

Masters and Johnson, in their pioneering work on the human sexual response, divided the whole sequence into four succes-

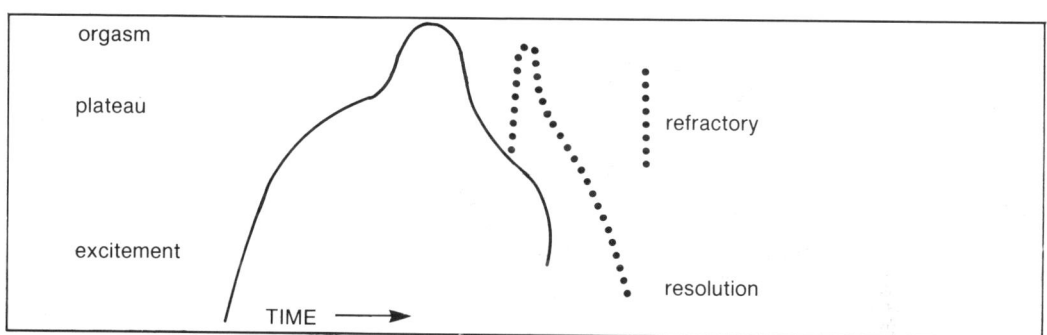

Sexual response in men

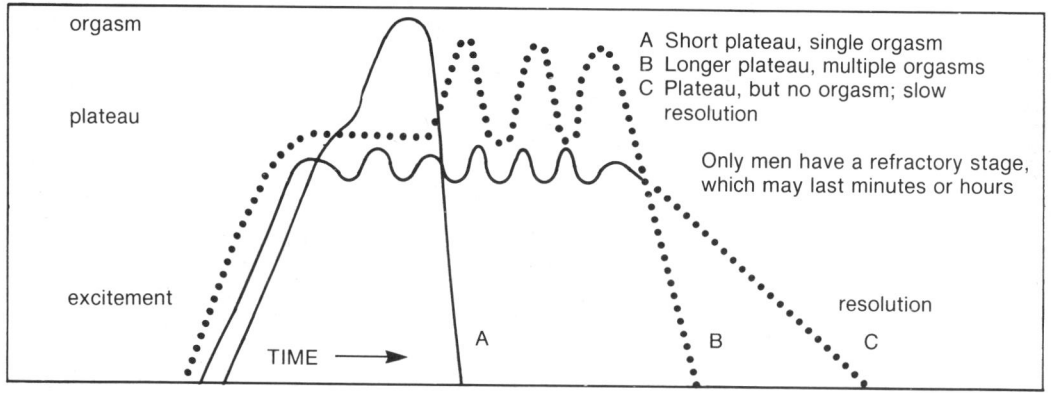

A Short plateau, single orgasm
B Longer plateau, multiple orgasms
C Plateau, but no orgasm; slow resolution

Only men have a refractory stage, which may last minutes or hours

Sexual response in women

43

sive stages. These are (1) the excitement stage, (2) the 'plateau' stage, (3) the orgasm stage, and (4) the resolution stage.

## Excitement stage

When a person is sexually excited more blood flows into the genital organs than flows out so that they become 'congested'; in other words they have more blood in them. A man's penis becomes hard and erect because there are valves which let the blood flow in and prevent it from flowing out. Often a drop of moisture may come out of the 'eye' of the penis. When erect, a man's penis doubles, or even more than doubles, its non-aroused length. The larger the penis when non-aroused, the less it increases in length, so that erect penises are generally about the same length. Their size, that is their circumference, may vary considerably. Some women are afraid that they may be damaged if a man with a large penis tries to insert it into the vagina. They believe that the vagina may be too small. It is never too small.

With increasing sexual excitement, a woman's vagina becomes increasingly moist as fluid seeps through its walls, and she begins to develop a softness at its entrance as the network of blood vessels in the tissue becomes congested with blood. The moisture, which is called vaginal lubrication, and the softness at its entrance will make sexual intercourse more pleasant.

## Plateau stage

Quickly or slowly, depending on the degree with which the 'sex centre' helps or hinders your response, you reach the plateau stage. By now the sexual tension is high, and the sexual enjoyment greater. In the plateau stage a man's penis is firmly erect. His testicles have increased in size and have been drawn up nearer to his crutch as the skin of his scrotum has become tighter.

A woman's vagina becomes increasingly wet and the swellings around the entrance to her vagina increase in size to become

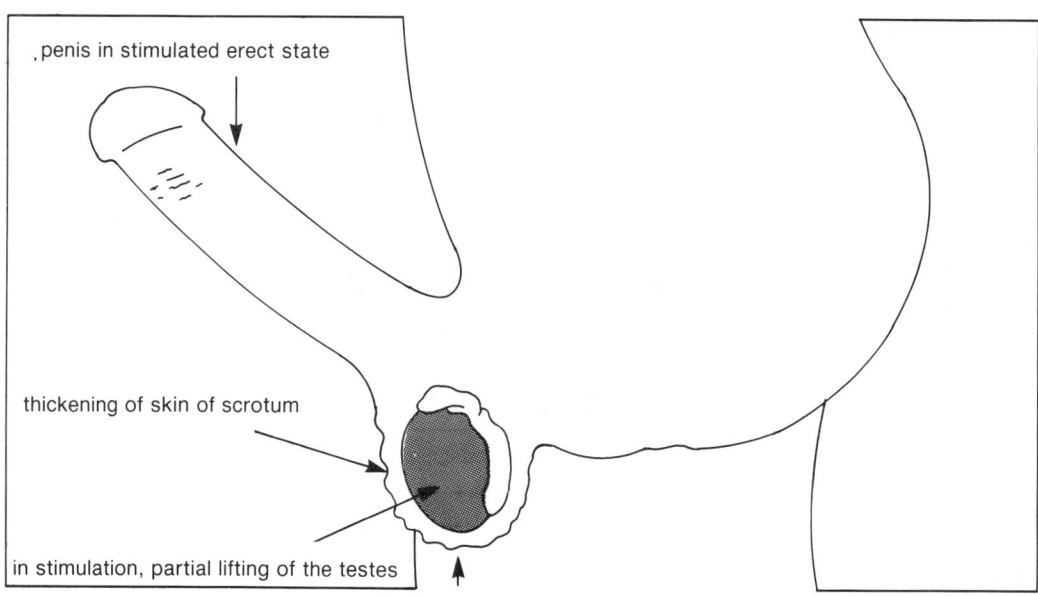

penis in stimulated erect state

thickening of skin of scrotum

in stimulation, partial lifting of the testes

Sexual response: excitement stage in a man

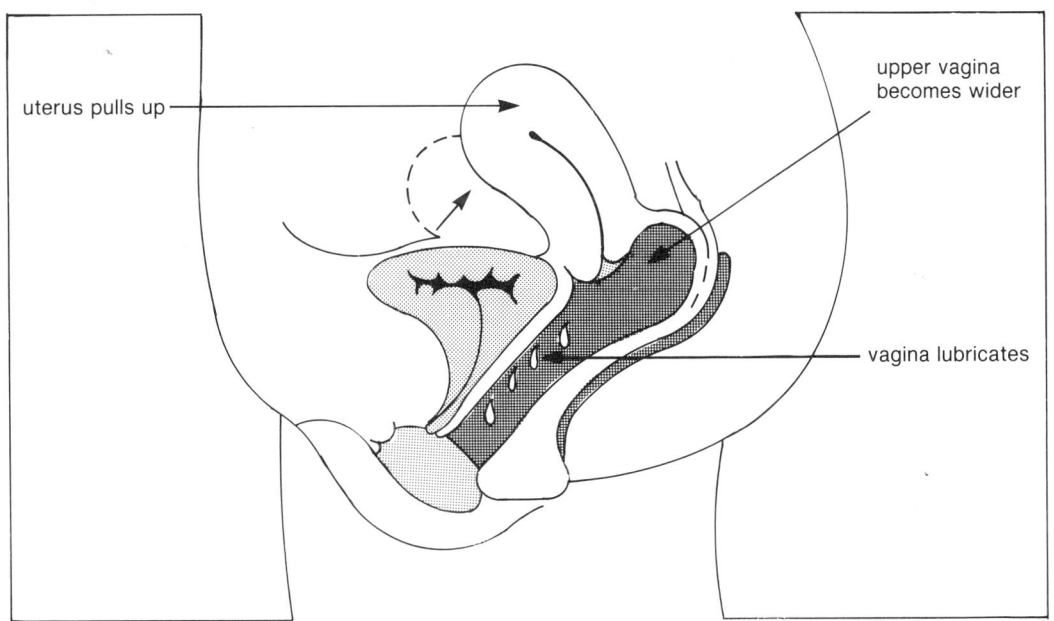

Sexual response: excitement stage in a woman

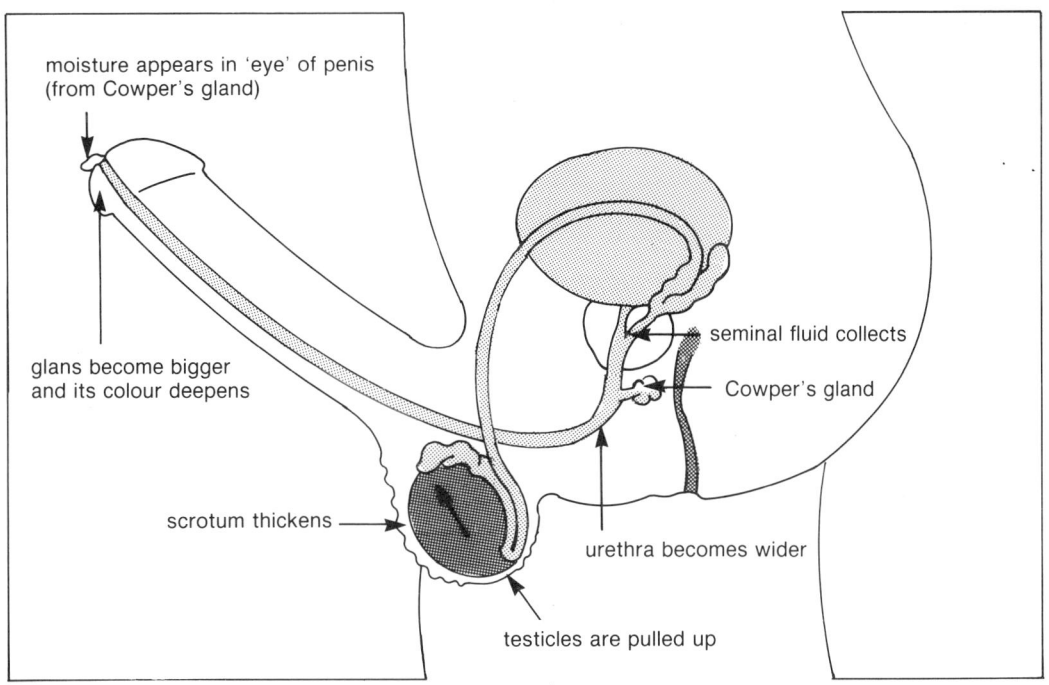

Sexual response: plateau stage in a man

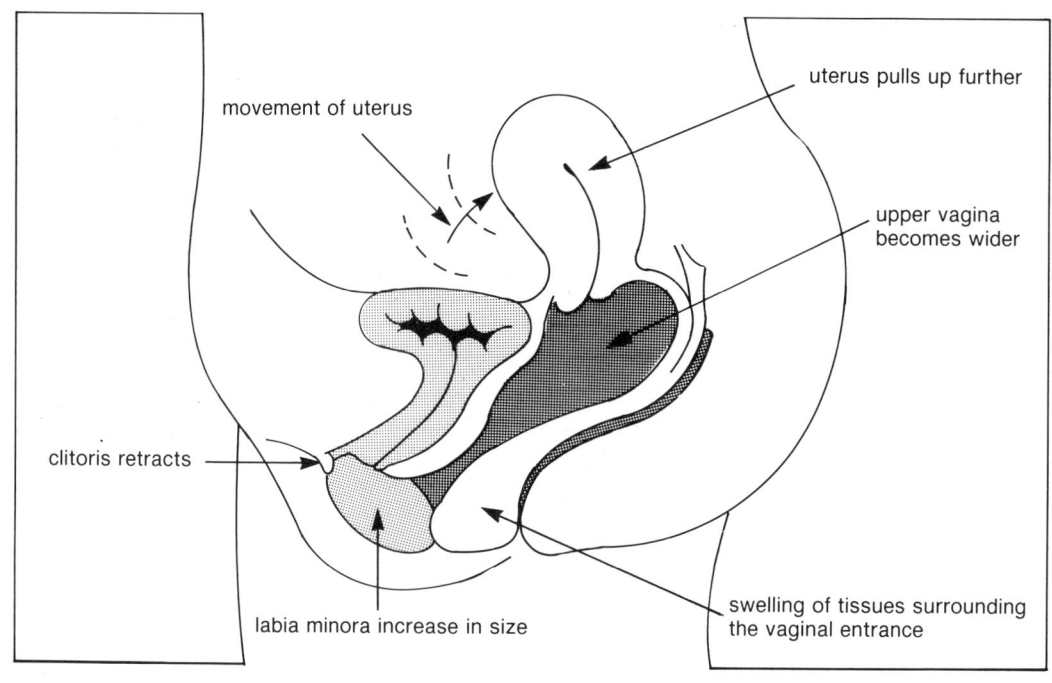

movement of uterus

uterus pulls up further

upper vagina becomes wider

clitoris retracts

labia minora increase in size

swelling of tissues surrounding the vaginal entrance

Sexual response: plateau stage in a woman

soft, moist, swollen 'sex cushions' which will caress the man's penis gently when it enters her vagina. To help this happen, her vaginal entrance opens slightly. At the same time her clitoris has drawn up under its hood and may have become almost hidden behind the pubic bone. The inner lips surrounding the vagina become increasingly dark red in colour.

The plateau stage can be very short, or it can be prolonged by lovers who are able to tell each other what pleasures them most so that both get the greatest enjoyment.

By now the man will probably want to insert his penis into the woman's vagina and she may want to feel it inside her body so that the couple can be as close as possible to each other. The woman may guide the man's penis with her hand or move her body so that it slips easily into her wet vagina.

As the man's penis moves within the woman's vagina, he reaches the stage when he knows that he is going to have an orgasm. When this stage is reached nothing can stop him from 'coming'.

## Orgasm phase

An orgasm is a deeply joyous sensation, which begins as a warm feeling deep in the pelvis and sweeps upwards and over the person's body so that it obliterates all other feelings and any preoccupations, worries or fears. It completely absorbs the person whilst it lasts, and when it goes it leaves behind a glow of pleasure, of relaxation, of togethernesss and of joy.

An orgasm is not the same as ejaculation, which is the spurting of sperm from a man's penis, although in most men orgasm and ejaculation occur together. A

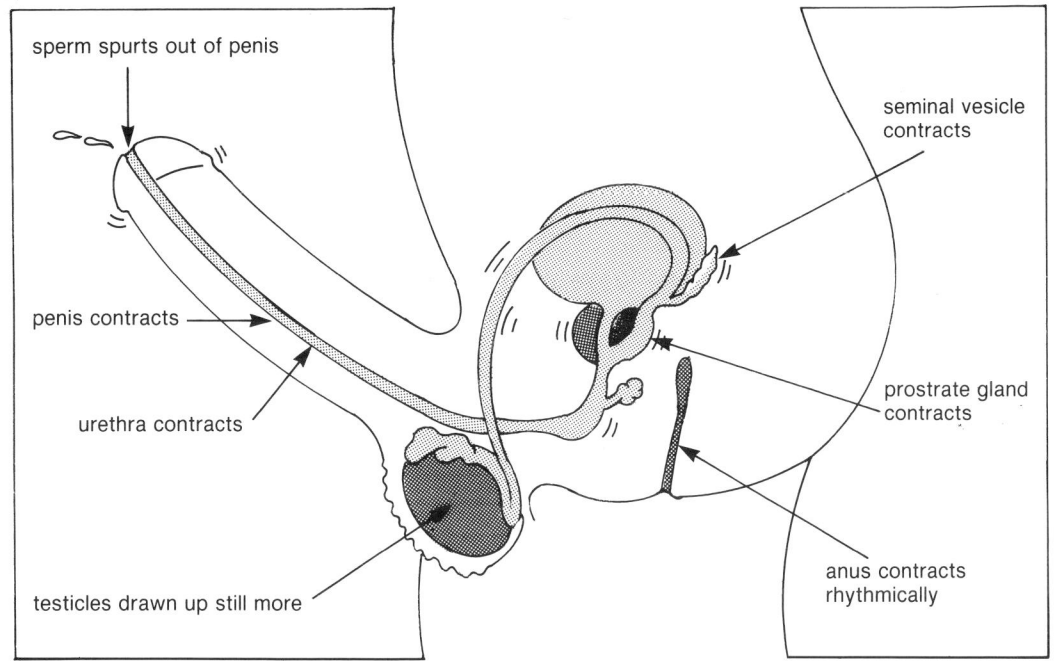

sperm spurts out of penis

seminal vesicle
contracts

penis contracts

urethra contracts

prostrate gland
contracts

anus contracts
rhythmically

testicles drawn up still more

Sexual response: orgasmic stage in a man

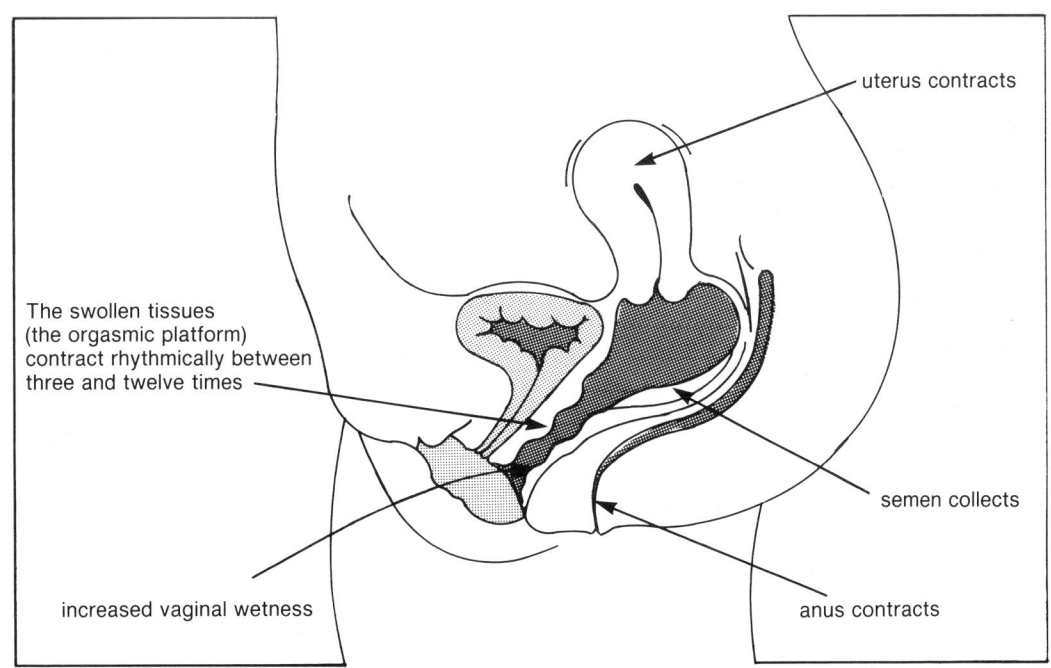

uterus contracts

The swollen tissues
(the orgasmic platform)
contract rhythmically between
three and twelve times

semen collects

increased vaginal wetness

anus contracts

Sexual response: orgasmic stage in a woman

woman doesn't ejaculate, but she has an orgasm, although she may not have it at the same time as the man.

As well as the sensation of orgasm, the muscles surrounding the base of a man's penis and a woman's vagina contract rhythmically at intervals of four-fifths of a second. A mild orgasm is accompanied by three to five contractions, a strong orgasm by eight to twelve; some orgasms are accompanied by up to twenty contractions. Other muscles also become involved and contract, so that an orgasm may be associated with contractions of the muscles of the back and the abdomen, with clutching hands, with grunting or with sighing, and sometimes with facial grimaces.

With the first contraction, semen is propelled along the man's urethra and spurts rhythmically until it has all been ejaculated. Semen is a mixture of sperm and the secre-

tions of the prostate gland and the seminal vesicles.

Each time a man has an orgasm, he ejaculates between 2 and 5 ml of semen (about a teaspoonful). The semen contains between 100 million and 500 million sperms.

Under a microscope the sperms look like tadpoles. They have a narrow snake-like head, a thickened area like a collar called the middle piece, which is the power-house for the sperm, and a long tail. They move by thrashing their tails. The head of the sperm contains the nucleus, and inside that are the twenty-three chromosomes, including an X or a Y sex chromosome.

Nearly every man has an orgasm when he ejaculates, although the intensity of the orgasm may vary from very strong to moderate. In contrast, only about half of all women have an orgasm whilst the man's

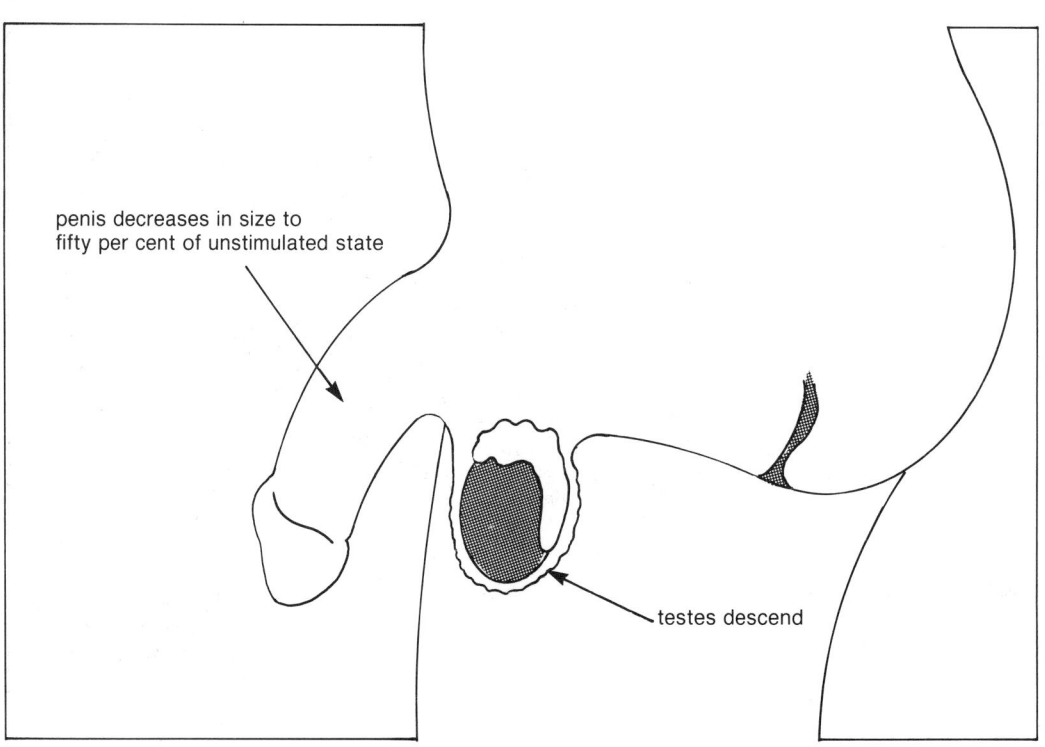

penis decreases in size to fifty per cent of unstimulated state

testes descend

Sexual response: resolution stage in a man

penis is thrusting in the vagina, but some of these women may have several orgasms in quick succession—something no man can do.

If the woman does not normally have an orgasm during sexual intercourse, a man who is a considerate lover can help her to have an orgasm before he does, or afterwards. Only she knows her own response and what stimulates her, and if the couple talk with each other the man will find out what her needs are. He can help her have an orgasm by stimulating her clitoris gently, at her direction, with his tongue or his moistened finger. Most women reach orgasm in this way, but some women take rather longer than others.

Sex is communication, sex is cooperation, sex is consideration of one's partner's needs.

## Resolution phase

And then it's over. The intense pleasure of the orgasm has passed, leaving a warm relaxed sensation as an afterglow. The couple may want to lie in each other's arms, their bodies in close contact, each enjoying the closeness, the touch and the smell of the other. Often they fall asleep in each other's arms, to wake after a short period, still entwined. During this period of time the blood which congested the genital organs drains away. The penis becomes

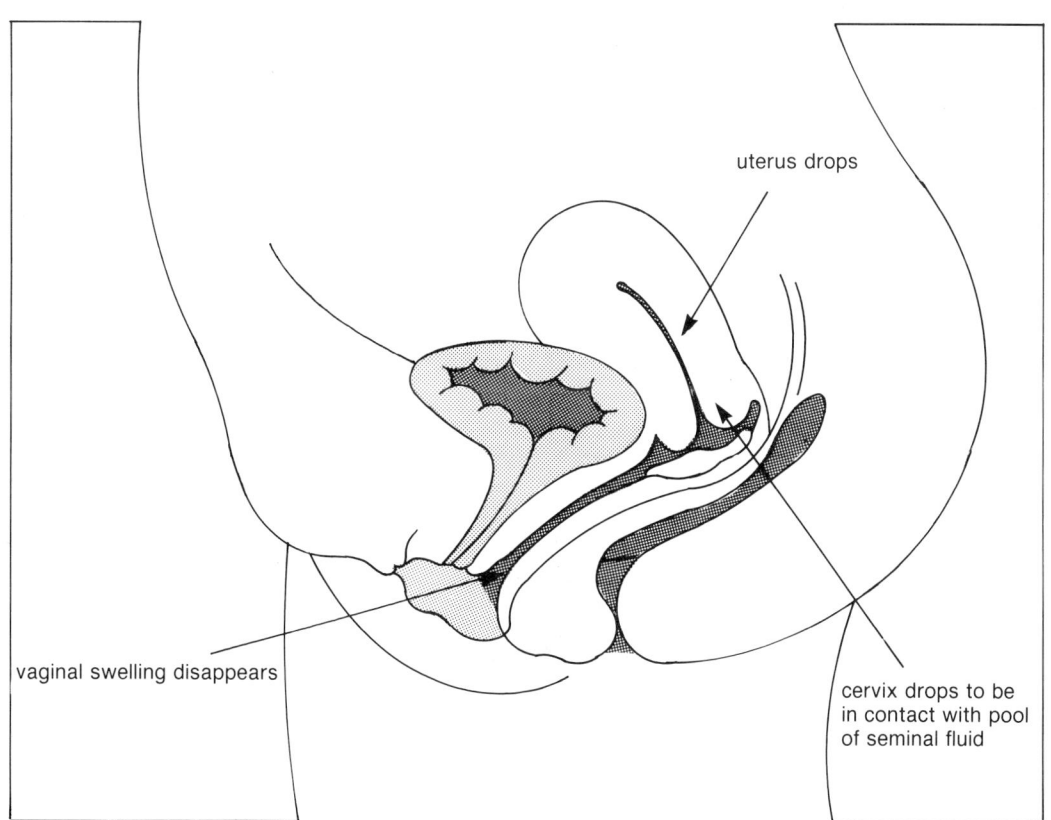

uterus drops

vaginal swelling disappears

cervix drops to be in contact with pool of seminal fluid

Sexual response: resolution stage in a woman

49

limp, the sex cushions disappear. The man is now in a stage when for many minutes or perhaps hours, he cannot become sexually aroused or get another erection. For some young men the period is quite short: some men can have another orgasm in five minutes; but most men need a longer interval, and as a man grows older, the refractory period lengthens.

By contrast, women have no refractory period. Many women, if effectively stimulated, can have a second orgasm with almost no interval, and then a third and fourth.

# People's sexual response varies

The sexual response often doesn't exactly follow the pattern described because each person is unique and responds uniquely to sexual arousal. Just as everybody has a face with two eyes, a mouth, a nose and two ears, but is different from everybody else, so every person responds sexually slightly differently, although everyone shows some of the responses described.

These responses occur whether the sexual arousal is brought about by heavy pet-

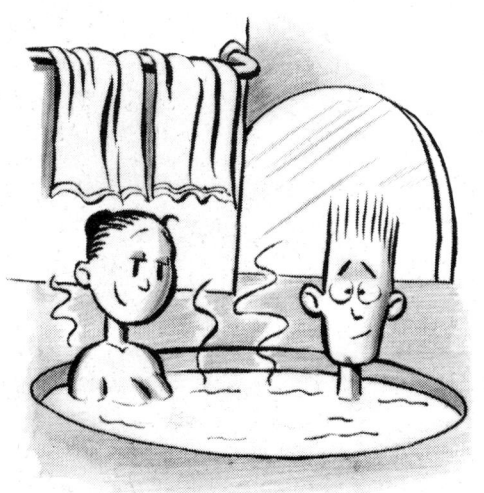

ting, by masturbation, during oral sex, or during sexual intercourse. Some people say that they get a more intense orgasm by masturbating, others that their most intensely pleasurable orgasm is from oral sex. Still others say that the orgasm from masturbation is not bad and that from oral sex is usually good, but the best orgasm comes from sexual intercourse, particularly when both partners are close, relaxed, and deeply in love.

# Touching is sex too

In our society, boys are brought up to believe that to touch another person is not mannish, and that to show emotion is 'sissy'. In other societies, it is normal and quite acceptable for people to show their emotions, and men and women are able to touch each other openly and without inhibition.

For many people the enjoyment of the excitement and plateau stages of the human sexual response is increased if the partners are able to explore each other's bodies with their fingers, their lips and their tongues, trying to find out what turns on the other person most.

Many women complain that their lovers are so anxious to have intercourse that they don't seem to want to spend time in touching and pleasuring their partner. This often reduces the woman's enjoyment of sex.

Unfortunately, many women don't tell their partners what they need so that they will enjoy sex more, nor do they find out what most pleasures the man. This criticism applies equally to men. Men often fail to find out what their partner likes most in love play, and don't tell their partner what they want most.

Sex is touching, and even more, sex is communicating your thoughts and feelings to your loved one.

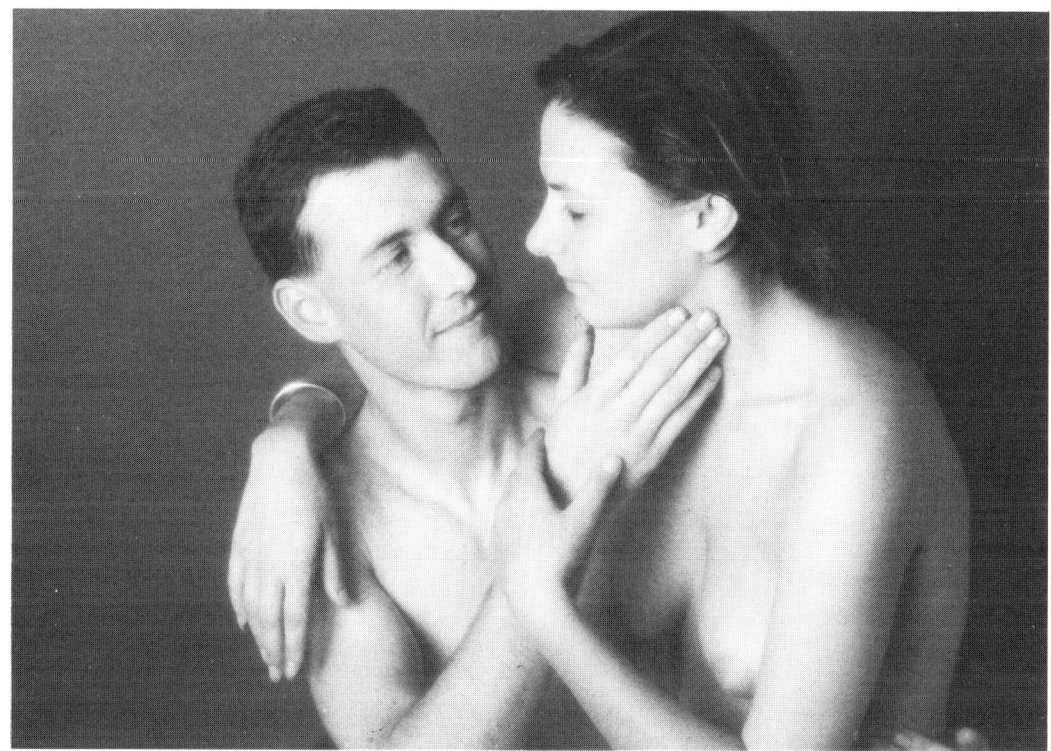
Touching is sex too

## Investigations
● Observe how people touch each other. What are some of the differences and similarities between the way in which (a) males and females, and (b) people from various cultural backgrounds, touch?

## Discussions
● What are some of the ways (besides sexual intercourse) in which partners may give sexual pleasure to each other?
● Communicating thoughts and feelings about sexuality can be very difficult. How do you think this could be made easier?

## Activities
● Make a table of the similarities and differences between males and females in the four stages of the sexual response cycle.
● Look at some magazines designed for women and for men. How do they emphasize
(a) sexual attractiveness?
(b) male and female expressions of sexuality?
(c) the provision of information about sexuality?
(d) response to readers' questions about sexuality?
● How accurate are these messages? How might they affect the readers?

# Myths about the sexual response

| Myth | Fact |
| --- | --- |
| • Men need sex more than women. | • Untrue. Women and men have similar sexual desires and needs. These vary between individuals, not between the sexes. |
| • Men are the sex experts who should always initiate sex. | • Untrue. |
| • A man needs 'to sow his wild oats' before marrying; a woman should remain a virgin. | • When a woman was believed to be a man's possession this view was acceptable. If a woman is a man's equal partner, either both should remain virgins or both should have equal opportunities for premarital sex. |
| • A man needs to have an orgasm to relieve his 'sexual tension'; a woman is content to have sex without an orgasm, to please her man. | • True, if you believe that women are sexually inferior. If you believe that women have equal sexual needs and rights to men, then it is false. |
| • The larger a man's penis, the better he is as a lover. | • The size of the penis has nothing to do with being a good lover. A good lover is considerate and tries to find out what makes his partner happiest. |
| • If a man doesn't have regular orgasms, his penis shrinks and his testicles become swollen and tender (blue balls). | • This is all complete nonsense. |

# 6

# FAMILY PLANNING

## A decision about sex

If your decision is that you will enjoy a sexual relationship with one or more partners, two consequences may occur. The first is that the woman may become unexpectedly pregnant. The second is that one or both of you may contract a sexually transmitted disease. Both these consequences can be avoided.

In this chapter I will discuss the available methods of birth control which can prevent an unwanted pregnancy from occurring.

In spite of the knowledge that contraception can prevent an unwanted pregnancy, a very large number of young teenaged women continue to become pregnant. Statistics from the USA showed that between 1983 and 1985, 825 000 American teenaged girls—that is 9 per cent of all adolescent women—became pregnant each year.

Four out of every five teenaged pregnancies occurred to unmarried teenaged women, and four out of five of them were not intended. So in four out of five cases the pregnancy was most probably unwelcome. Of those who became pregnant few used reliable contraceptives.

This is irresponsible, for sexual intercourse without contraceptive protection is likely to lead to pregnancy. In spite of this, several American surveys show that only thirty per cent of unmarried teenaged women, or their male friend, used reliable contraceptives each time they had sexual intercourse at least in the first six months of being sexually active. This pattern is repeated in Great Britain, in Australia, in New Zealand, and in other countries, judging by the numbers of unintended pregnancies which occur.

## Why are contraceptives not used?

It is not clear why so many sexually active couples fail to use reliable contraceptives or any contraceptive at all. There are many possible reasons. One is said to be that in many cases the boy and girl didn't intend to have sexual intercourse, but 'got carried away'. Another reason is that some girls don't want to use contraceptives because that would make them seem to be planning to have sex, and they want to believe it happens spontaneously. A few girls have sex to *become* pregnant, perhaps because they want to escape from, or hurt, parents they don't get on with, or because they believe the boy will have to marry a girl who is pregnant, and they believe themselves to be in love.

Most pregnancies, it seems, occur because of lack of information about contraceptives, a false modesty about using them, or difficulty in obtaining them.

The information about the sexual activity of teenagers given earlier shows that increasing numbers are going to have sex-

# There are nine methods of birth control.

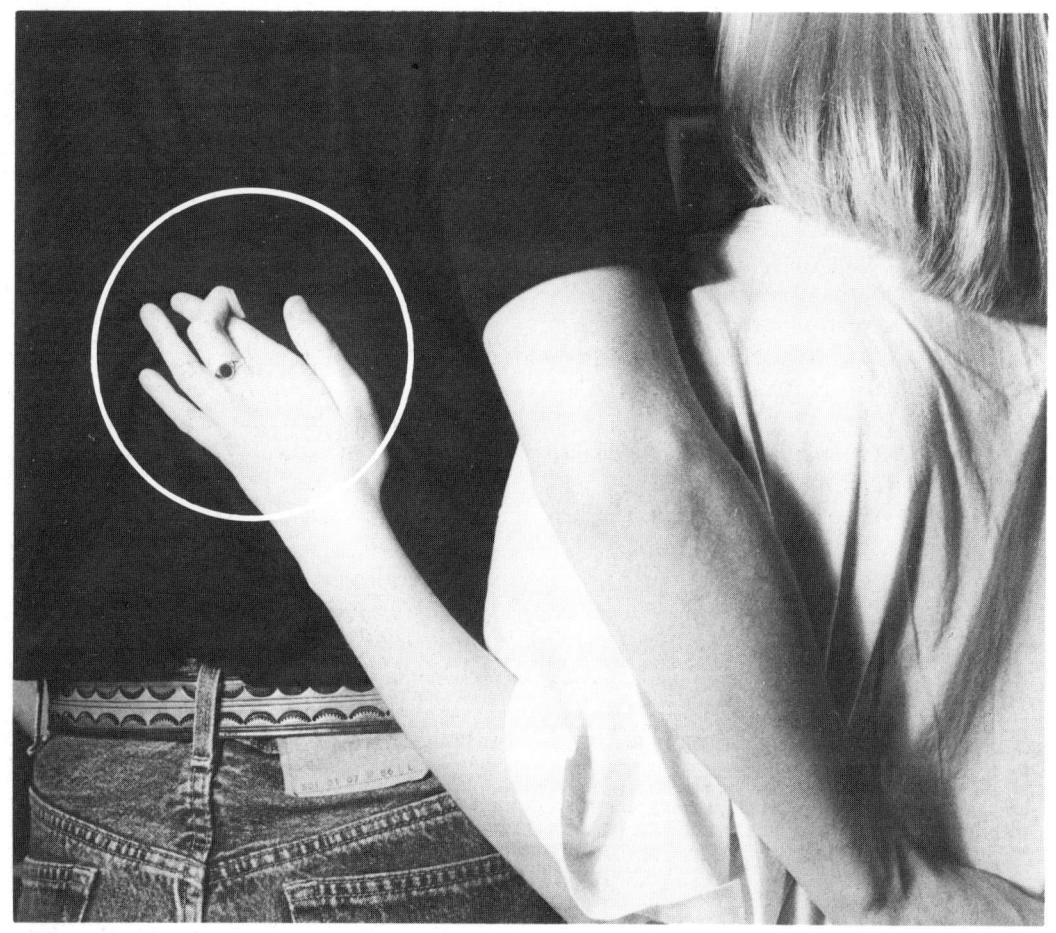

# This isn't one of them.

ual intercourse. So it is extremely important to know how to prevent conception and pregnancy—this knowledge can be made available to teenagers by society, by parents, by teachers, by doctors. There will be fewer unintended pregnancies only if most sexually active teenagers know about contraceptives and are able to obtain them and use them properly.

Some adults argue that this knowledge will lead to promiscuity. There is no evidence that this occurs. On the other hand, there is evidence that, without the use of contraception, large numbers of young unmarried women will become pregnant and will have an abortion induced, or will give birth to a baby born out of wedlock, or will enter a forced marriage.

Abortions are emotionally traumatic events, and usually are only sought after the woman has given considerable thought to the matter. Even in a society which provides help for single mothers, the problems she may encounter are considerable. And at least one-quarter of marriages between teenagers fail if the girl became pregnant before the marriage took place.

These undesirable and traumatic events could be avoided if contraception was used by every sexually active teenager who did not intend to become pregnant.

# What is contraception?

Contraception (or family planning) is any way of preventing the sperm from meeting the ovum, when the couple want to avoid a pregnancy.

You shouldn't confuse contraception with abortion, which is the interruption of a pregnancy that has already started.

Obviously it is better to prevent a pregnancy from occurring, rather than having to interrupt the pregnancy. That is why this chapter stresses contraception.

Obviously the most effective form of contraception is for a woman to say NO—and mean it!—when a man asks, or tries to have sex with her. But many couples enjoy making love. They should choose which method of contraception is most appropriate for their particular needs. Unless they agree that the man will use a condom, it means going to a Family Planning Clinic or to a doctor for advice. Many young women prefer to go to a Family Planning Clinic as the people there are usually women and seem more sympathetic than some doctors. When the choices of contraception available have been discussed, a couple can make an intelligent, informed decision.

Many young women are able to tell their parents that they are having sex and have decided to use contraceptives. But some young women feel that their parents would be outraged and angry if they knew that their daughter was having sex. If the young woman proposes to disregard her parents' views on sex, it is better she should obtain contraceptives than risk becoming pregnant. This applies to women under the age of sixteen—the age of consent. It is not a crime for the woman to have sex, nor is it a crime for her to be given contraception, although the young man who has sex with her is committing a crime.

If you are to use contraception properly you must know the methods available and be able to choose and use the one which suits your needs most exactly. The main methods are shown in the table. They are:

**Mechanical methods**, which prevent the sperm from reaching the ovum
• Condoms for use by the man
• Vaginal diaphragms for use by the woman

**Hormonal contraception**, which prevents the ovum from developing in and escaping from the ovary
• The Pill

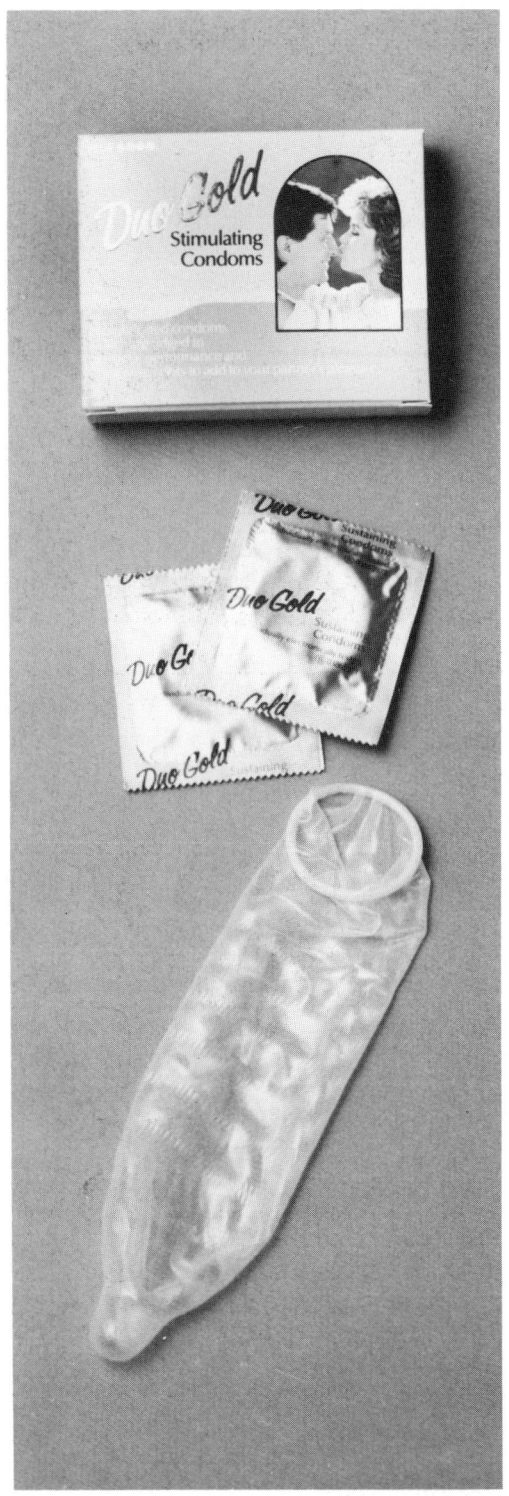

**Intrauterine devices**, which prevent the sperm from reaching the ovum at the right time, or perhaps prevent the fertilized egg from implanting into the uterus
• The IUD

**Period abstinence** (called the rhythm method, the ovulation method, or the mucus method). In this method the couple avoid intercourse at the time of ovulation and for two or three days each side of it. As the egg and the sperm only live to two or three days, pregnancy is avoided.

# Condoms

The first condom is said to have been used in Roman times. It was made of sheep's intestine and was not very satisfactory. Modern condoms are made of thin but strong latex rubber, and are scarcely noticed when placed on the man's erect penis; they do not reduce the pleasurable sensations of sexual intercourse. Today you can buy condoms in different colours which turn some people on.

Condoms can be purchased from chemists, and from vending machines. They are packed in sealed foil packs, which keeps the latex in good condition until the man wants to use the condom. When a condom has been used once it is discarded.

Most condoms are prelubricated with a sperm-killing jelly, which makes them easy to draw onto the penis and helps to prevent any live sperms escaping into the woman's vagina should the condom tear or slip off the man's penis after he has ejaculated.

Condoms are made with teat ends and plain ends. There isn't much difference between the two. Both kinds must be unrolled onto the man's erect penis making sure that there is no air bubble at the end, because the pressure of air together with the semen may burst the condom. A condom must also be unrolled fully so that it reaches down the length of the penis; otherwise, after ejaculation when the man's penis becomes small, the condom may slip off and release the sperms in the woman's vagina. A condom is a most appropriate contraceptive when sexual intercourse only takes place infrequently.

Provided it is placed on the penis properly and used each time a man has sexual intercourse, a condom is a very reliable method of preventing an unwanted pregnancy.

Condoms are also the only effective way, apart from abstaining from sex, of reducing the spread of sexually transmitted diseases, including AIDS.

If you don't know the sexual behaviour of your partner, male or female, and intend to have sexual intercourse, it is important that the man wears a condom during the whole sex act.

Because males are more likely to have had a previous sexual partner than are females, many doctors now recommend that women and girls have a condom available and only permit sex if the man agrees to wear it.

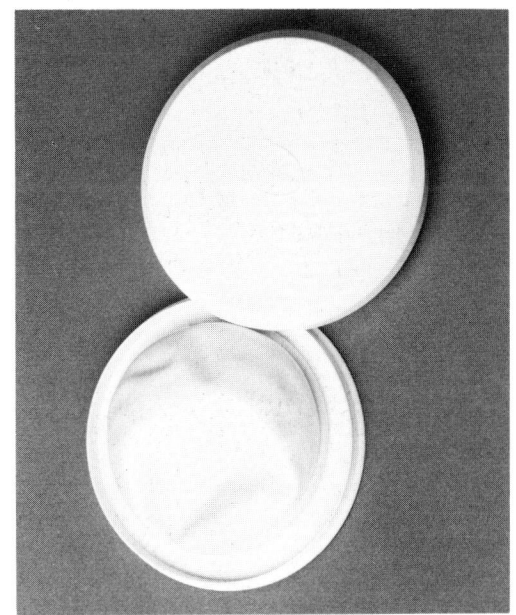

## Vaginal diaphragm

Between 1925 and 1965 the vaginal diaphragm was a popular method of birth control, particularly amongst middle-class women. With the introduction of the Pill the diaphragm lost favour, but it is now returning as its value is appreciated. The reason why few working-class women used the diaphragm was because the sexual modesty of the time demanded that a woman place the diaphragm in position in her vagina in private, which was often impossible.

Today diaphragms are making a comeback, and women are putting them into their vaginas either in private or with their partner's help during love play.

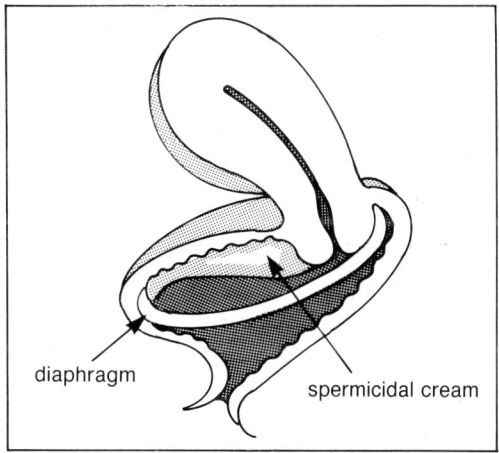

diaphragm                    spermicidal cream

The diaphragm consists of a thin rubber dome which has a flexible 'arcing' spring in its edge. This enables a woman to squeeze it so that she can place it in her vagina easily, knowing it will regain its shape when it is inside.

Spermicidal cream should be smeared around the rim of the diaphragm and placed in its dome, so that it rubs onto the woman's cervix.

The diaphragm works by preventing the sperms from reaching the cervix, leaving them in the vagina where they are killed by the vaginal acidity.

If a woman decides to use a diaphragm she must be examined vaginally by a doctor and the appropriate size for her chosen. Once she has become used to introducing the diaphragm into her vagina properly, neither she nor her partner will notice its presence when they have sexual intercourse.

The woman keeps the diaphragm in her vagina for at least 6 hours after the last time she makes love, and then takes it out. She should wash it, dry it carefully, powder it lightly, and place it in its plastic box until she wants to use it again.

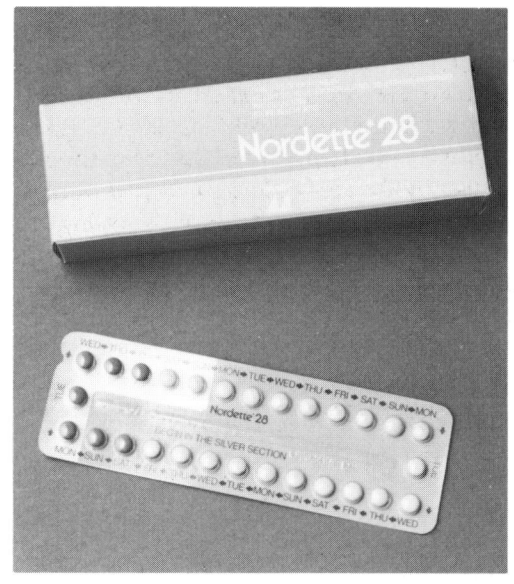

# The hormonal contraceptives—the Pill

More women today use the Pill than any other method to prevent pregnancy. No drug (and it is a drug) has been investigated more fully than the Pill. It is the most efficient way of protecting a woman from an unwanted pregnancy, apart from abstaining from sexual intercourse.

The Pill works by preventing the egg from developing and being pushed out of the ovary. It also changes the nature of the secretions of the cervix so that sperms find it difficult to penetrate them and it alters the lining of the uterus so that it is not suitable to receive an egg, should one escape from the ovary.

The Pill is composed of two hormones made in the laboratory. They are **oestrogen** and **progestogen** (a laboratory-produced hormone resembling progesterone). The oestrogen prevents ovulation occurring, the progestogen makes the secretions of the cervix tacky and alters the lining of the uterus. It also regulates the

menstrual period which occurs when a woman uses the Pill. Both hormones are necessary. The original Pill had much larger doses of hormones than today's Pill. In the Pill prescribed today, the amount of the hormones is quite low, and this has made the Pill very safe.

Most of the Pills available today are pre-packed in plastic and it is easy to follow the instructions. The packs usually have twenty-eight pills, of which twenty-one contain the hormones and seven are sugar pills. It is usual to start taking the tablets on the first day of menstruation (day 1) and to follow the sequence on the package. It is important to remember to take a tablet every day as nearly as possible at the same time each day. If you forget to take the tablet and more than twelve hours have passed, another method of contraception, such as a condom, should be used until the package is completed. For complete protection it is wise for the man to use a condom during the first month the woman takes the Pill.

It is known today that a woman can continue taking the Pill for years with safety, provided she has regular check-ups from a doctor. The Pill has some side-effects; some women are more affected by these than others. In the first month of using it some women feel nauseated, but this usually ceases by the second month. A few women find that from time to time 'spotting' of blood occurs. This is of no significance, but if the bleeding becomes heavier a doctor should be consulted.

# Intrauterine devices— the IUD

An intrauterine device is a small piece of polythene, sometimes with fine copper wire twisted around its stem. The plastic has a 'memory'. When the IUD is stretched into a narrow tube, so that it can be introduced easily into the uterus, it keeps its memory. When it is pushed into the uterus it regains its previous shape.

The IUD works partly by preventing the sperm wriggling through the uterus and partly by so altering the lining of the uterus that the egg can't implant.

Usually it is chosen as a contraceptive by a woman who has had a baby, because then it is easier to put into her uterus. The new smaller IUDs can be used for women who have never been pregnant, but should be avoided by most women who have not had a baby because the IUD increases her risk of developing pelvic infection. This may reduce her chance of becoming pregnant later when she wants to have a baby.

An IUD is put in in the doctor's surgery, and usually you don't need an anaesthetic. The best time to have it put in your uterus is at the end of a menstrual period. You may feel a little discomfort, or a bit faint, during the procedure, but in most cases this passes very quickly. A few women bleed for a day or two after the IUD has

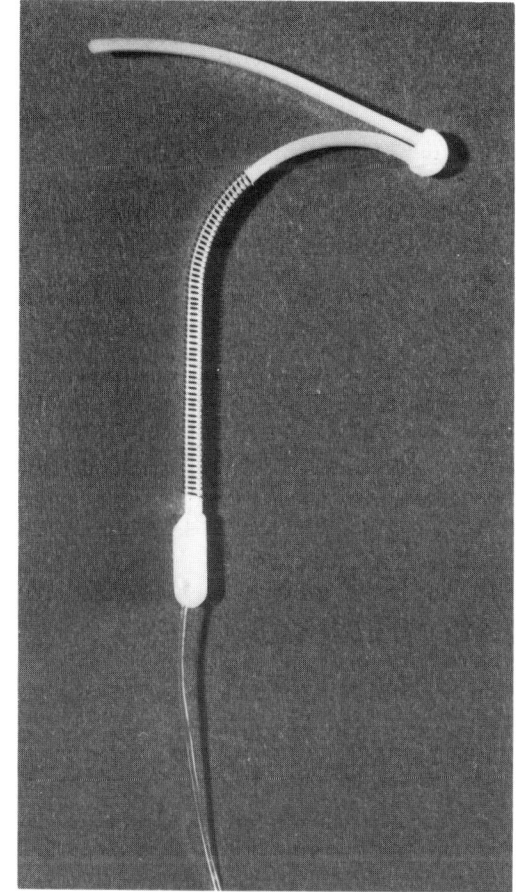

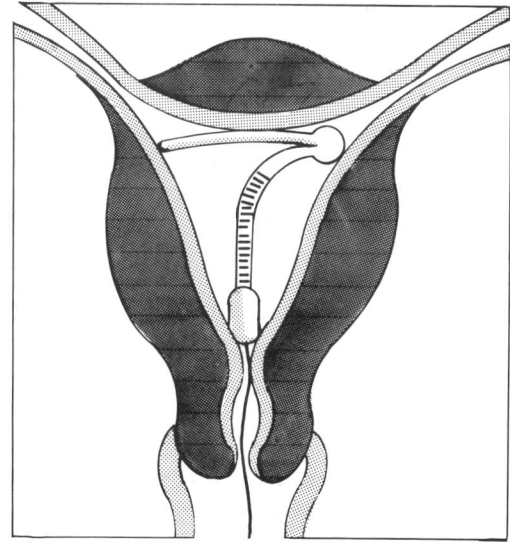

The IUD in position

59

been put in the uterus, but the bleeding is not usually heavy. The first one or two menstrual periods may be heavier than usual, but this usually settles down quite quickly.

A very few women who have an IUD get a heavy vaginal discharge and pain deep inside the pelvis, especially after sexual intercourse. If this happens the woman must see a doctor as she may have an infection in her pelvis.

A disadvantage of the diaphragm, the Pill and the IUD is that you have to go to the doctor or to a Family Planning Clinic to obtain them. Many sexually active teenaged girls are reluctant to do this; they are too shy to go or they believe they may be criticized for having sex. Most Family Planning Clinics have very sympathetic staffs (usually women) so if a girl is about to have sex and she wants to prevent a pregnancy, she need have no fear of or shame about seeing a counsellor in a Family Planning Clinic or a sympathetic, sensible doctor.

# Periodic abstinence

Most women find these methods inconvenient, and they are less reliable than other forms of birth control. Periodic abstinence methods include the 'calendar method' (in which the woman charts her menstrual cycle over six months and works out her 'safe' day), the 'temperature method' (in which she takes her temperature each morning when she wakes up, to give her an idea when she will ovulate) and the 'mucus' or 'ovulation method' (in which she checks each morning to find if she has any wetness in the entrance of her vagina).

Periodic abstinence is the only contraceptive method permitted by the Roman Catholic Church.

If the woman and her partner are motivated and follow the methods faithfully,

few pregnancies should occur. But many pregnancies do, because with these methods the couple can only have sexual intercourse at certain times, and the desire to have sexual intercourse may be almost overpoweringly strong at the wrong times, that is, when the woman is ovulating, sometime around the middle of the menstrual cycle. Periodic abstinence requires motivation, discipline and devotion if it is to be used successfully.

# Induced abortion

In a sense an abortion, that is the termination, induced by a doctor, of a pregnancy before the twentieth week, is a form of birth control (but not of contraception). Abortion is discussed in the next chapter.

# Risks associated with pregnancy

Pregnancy in teenagers, especially young teenagers (that is, women aged sixteen or less), carries greater risk than pregnancy in women aged from twenty to thirty. The main problems are that more teenaged expectant mothers are anaemic or develop a raised blood pressure in pregnancy. These problems and others increase the chance that the birth weight of the baby will be low. In fact, mothers aged nineteen or less are one and a half times more likely to give birth to a low-birth-weight baby than mothers aged between twenty and twenty-nine. Low birth weight increases the chance that the baby will die; and there is a higher perinatal mortality (the deaths of babies around the time of birth) among babies born to teenaged mothers.

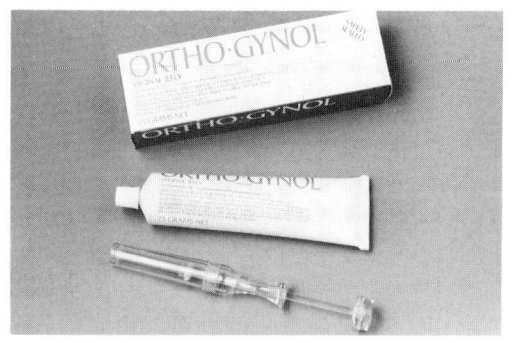

# Unreliable, or unsuitable, methods of contraception

Other forms of contraception are available, and unfortunately are often used by teenagers. They are not reliable in preventing an unintended pregnancy.

## Withdrawal (coitus interruptus)

This is not reliable as the man has to withdraw his penis from the woman's vagina before ejaculation. This requires timing, concentration, and agility. Often one of the three is lacking and some sperms spurt into the vagina.

## Vaginal spermicidal foams, tablets or creams

These are sometimes used; they are quite unreliable when used alone. But, if the man is using a condom, or the woman is using a diaphragm, the additional use of one of the vaginal spermicides gives an added protection.

## Injectables

A few doctors give an injection of hormones every three months, but these are not suitable for teenagers in general as the woman is unable to become pregnant for a period of about a year after the last injection.

## Permanent methods of birth control

These consist of tying the woman's oviducts or the man's vas, and are not appropriate for teenagers, who have either not started a family or may wish to have another child at some time in the future.

# How effective are the contraceptives?

If you look at pages 63 and 64 you can work out for yourself which of the contraceptive methods are the most effective. If you are sexually active and a responsible person, you will make sure that you don't have sexual intercourse unless you or your partner is protected against an unwanted pregnancy.

If you are a girl, it is stupid to believe the boy if he says it will be 'all right'. It almost certainly won't, unless he has a condom and wears it properly on his penis. Don't forget that you get pregnant, not him.

If you are a boy and you want sex, it is irresponsible to have sexual intercourse unless the girl really wants it too, and either you use a condom or she is using a contraceptive. If neither of you are using contraceptives, wait, don't risk making the girl pregnant. Pregnancy has three outcomes: you marry and have a baby born in wedlock. You don't marry and the girl has a baby born out of wedlock, which she brings up as a single mother or has adopted. Both of these eventualities may be very traumatic for a teenaged girl. Finally, the girl, her parents, or you may decide she should have an abortion. That is what we will discuss in the next chapter.

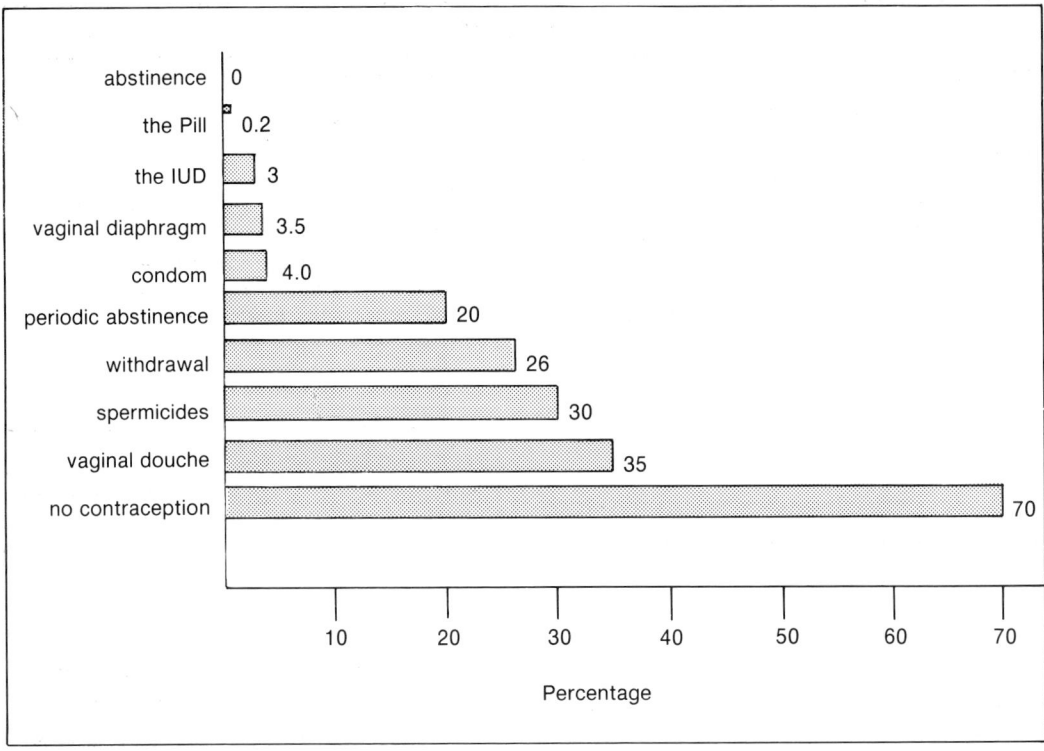

The chance of becoming pregnant in one year
using various methods of contraception

*Investigations*
● Examine some of the ways in which nature controls population, both for animals and for humans, while ensuring the continuation of the species.
● What are some of the attitudes towards birth control/family planning that you are aware of?
(a) How are the attitudes evident in our society?
(b) Are attitudes different in other countries?
(c) Have attitudes changed over the past ten, fifty years?
(d) Can you suggest any reasons for the changes you find?

*Discussions*
● In a sexual relationship, do you think one partner is more responsible for contraception than the other, or do you think the responsibility lies equally with both partners?
● Discuss the results of increasing acceptance and use of birth control and of the widespread introduction of more reliable methods.

*Activities*
● Obtain some samples of different contraceptive devices. Find out about their functions, method of use, and composition.

# Condoms

**Advantage**

- Harmless to either partner.
- Can be bought in chemist's shops and from slot machines without a doctor's prescription.
- Are pre-lubricated with spermicide and can be put on easily.
- Protect against sexually transmitted diseases.
- Readily available if you and your partner decide to have sex.

**Disadvantages**

- Have to be put on properly.
- Can only be used once.
- May tear, releasing sperms, unless care is taken.
- May slip off the penis when it becomes small after ejaculation. If the penis is still in the vagina, sperms may escape.

# Diaphragm

**Advantages**

- Has no side-effects.
- Is cheap, and can be used for up to two years.
- Possibly is a protection against cancer of the cervix of the uterus.
- Is very efficient in protecting a woman against pregnancy.

**Disadvantages**

- Requires some knowledge of anatomy and some skill in positioning it properly.
- Needs to be placed in the vagina before sexual arousal, or early in love-making.
- Needs to remain in the vagina for at least six hours after the last time the partner ejaculates.

# IUD

**Advantages**

- Once it is in your uterus you don't have to worry about it—you are protected.
- You don't have to remember to put in a diaphragm every time you have sex, or to take the Pill every day.

**Disadvantages**

- Some women get crampy pains at period times, and some get heavy periods.
- It has to be changed every two years or so.
- It is sometimes expelled. That is why it has a thread. You should examine your vagina to feel the thread from time to time— especially after your period.

# The Pill

## Advantages

- The most efficient method of preventing pregnancy—if you can remember to **take it every day**.

- Easy to carry about and to take.

- Stops cramping with the periods.

- Reduces the amount of menstrual flow, which may change in colour to red-brown rather than red.

## Disadvantages

- Some nausea in the first month.

- Some increase in vaginal discharge.

- Probably not suitable for women who have irregular or very light periods. They should choose another method of contraception.

- You have to go to a doctor (or a Family Planning Clinic) to get the Pill.

# Myths about the Pill

## Myth

- It leads to promiscuity. It makes you want and need sex often.

- You should stop the Pill for a month or two every three years to let your ovaries recover.

- If you take the Pill before you marry you will not be able to have a baby.

- The Pill is dangerous.

## Fact

- It doesn't.

- If you do you'll probably get pregnant—and there is no medical evidence that you should stop the Pill.

- False. Most women become pregnant within three months of stopping the Pill.

- Women over thirty-five, who are overweight, and who smoke heavily, have a **slightly** increased risk of having a clot in a vein, or a stroke.
  Teenagers are not at risk.

# 7
# ABORTION

Abortion is the termination (ending) of a pregnancy before the fetus is able to survive independently outside its mother's uterus. In general this time is accepted as being before the end of the twentieth week of pregnancy, when the fetus weighs about 500 g. Abortion means either that the fetus is expelled by nature, when it is called a spontaneous abortion (or a miscarriage), or that it is removed by a doctor (or some other person), because of disease or because the woman doesn't want to continue with the pregnancy. Then it is called an induced abortion or a medical termination of pregnancy.

Until recently induced abortion was prohibited by law in most countries, although millions of women had abortions induced, either by trying to terminate the pregnancy themselves, or by going to a 'back street' abortionist or, if they were wealthy, to a doctor.

Now, in many nations, the laws relating to abortion have been relaxed considerably, and many women can have an abortion without risk of breaking the law.

This change has occurred for several reasons. First, it was realized that the law was constantly broken, many women having abortions even in countries where the law was strict. Second, the law discriminated against the poor. Wealthy women have always been able to find a competent, discreet, if expensive, doctor who would terminate the pregnancy for them. Poor women, without the resource of money or knowledge, had to go to 'back street' abortionists who were often incompetent, with

the result that the abortion was performed badly. As a result, many poor women died from bleeding or from infection. Third, there was an increasing awareness that until the fetus could survive apart from the mother, it could be considered as part of her body.

In countries which have relaxed their abortion laws, abortion is not available on demand but permitted if, in the opinion of a qualified doctor, the continuation of pregnancy would cause physical or emotional damage to the woman's health and well-being. It has been found that when the law has been changed the number of infected, septic, dangerous abortions has declined dramatically, as has the number of women dying after abortion. This is because the abortions are done in appropriately designed, equipped and staffed clinics or in hospitals, instead of being performed in secret, in inappropriate places.

The change in the law in most Western nations has not been without controversy.

At one extreme, the Roman Catholic Church and, to a lesser degree, the Protestant churches, have condemned the change. Roman Catholics argue that human life begins the moment the sperm fertilizes the egg. The fertilized egg reaches the uterus within four days, and implants in its lining. They say that any person who seeks to abort the fertilized egg is destroying human life—in other words murdering a human being, however small it is. They believe that abortion should be prohibited by law. A few theologians have argued that until the fertilized egg becomes recognizably human it is only *biological* life, not *human* life. This change occurs at about the tenth week of pregnancy, calculating this from the first day of the last menstrual period. They argue that early abortion (before the tenth week) is permissible.

At the other extreme, certain women's groups argue that as the fertilized egg, which develops into the fetus, cannot survive outside the mother's body, it should be considered part of her body, and she should have the right to choose whether to continue with the pregnancy or not. These groups want abortion on demand.

If a teenaged girl finds that she is pregnant because she or her partner failed to use contraceptives (or used them incorrectly), she has to make a decision. She has to decide whether to have the baby or to have an abortion. It is not an easy decision. She may be influenced by her family, by the man and perhaps by the man's family. She—or her parents—may feel that she is too young or too immature to bear and rear a baby. Neither she nor her parents may wish her to marry the man. The man may refuse to marry her. Her parents may be concerned about the attitudes of the neighbours to her pregnancy. They may feel that the family is shamed by it.

A girl in this situation needs helpful counselling and should obtain this—from some responsible person she knows and trusts or from a Family Planning Clinic—before she makes a decision about what to do. If she decides to have an abortion it must be *her* decision, however young she is.

There is some urgency; a decision must be made as soon as is possible. Medical evidence shows that an abortion is safest, is attended by the fewest side effects and is least stressing mentally, if it is done before

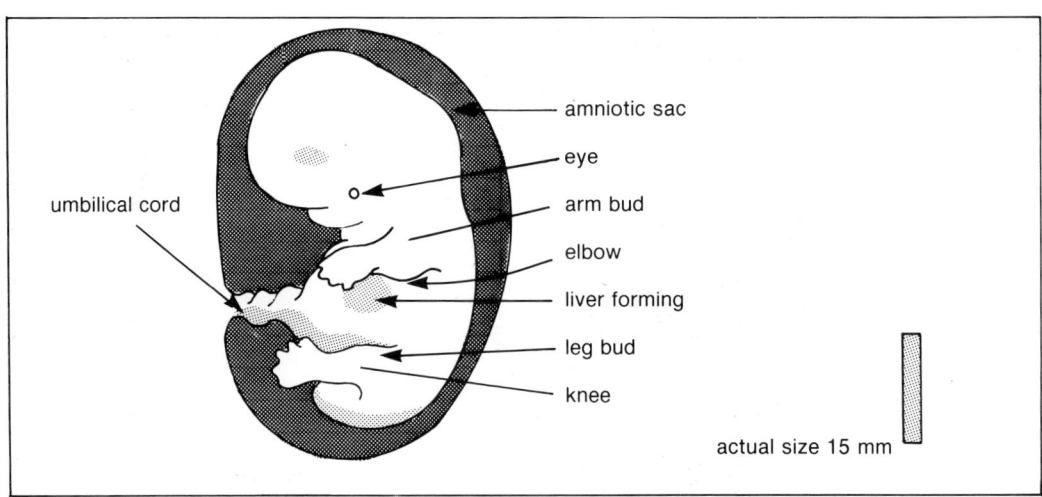

The embryo at 6 weeks after conception (8 weeks after the last menstrual period). It floats in the amniotic sac. Its eyes are open because the eyelids have not formed. Its limb buds are developing into arms and legs.

the end of the twelfth week after the last menstrual period, and preferably between the sixth and tenth week.

At this time the fetus is small. The smaller the fetus, the easier is the abortion. A girl who thinks she may be pregnant should not hide the pregnancy. If she usually has regular periods and her period is two to three weeks overdue she should tell her parents (if she feels she is able to). She should have a pregnancy test performed by a pharmacist or at a Family Planning Clinic, or she should visit a doctor, for the pregnancy to be diagnosed.

If the test is positive, she has to decide what to do. If she decides to have an abortion, this should be arranged with the least delay.

The abortion may be done in a special clinic or a hospital. Many of the special clinics, which don't look a bit like a hospital, are staffed entirely by women. The girl is encouraged to talk over her problem and to share her anxieties, her fears and her uncertainties with a trained counsellor, who will give her sympathetic help. If she still wants to have the abortion, she is seen by a doctor and the abortion is performed, either the same day or within a few days. When the abortion is performed, she is given a local anaesthetic injection into the cervix or, if she is in a hospital, she may have a general anaesthetic.

When the uterus is numb (anaesthetized), a narrow hollow plastic tube is pushed through the cervix so that it lies in the cavity of the uterus. This is connected to a small machine and the lining of the uterus, together with the tiny fetus and the small placenta, is sucked away from its attachment to the inside of the uterus.

The operation takes less than five minutes, and after it the woman remains in the

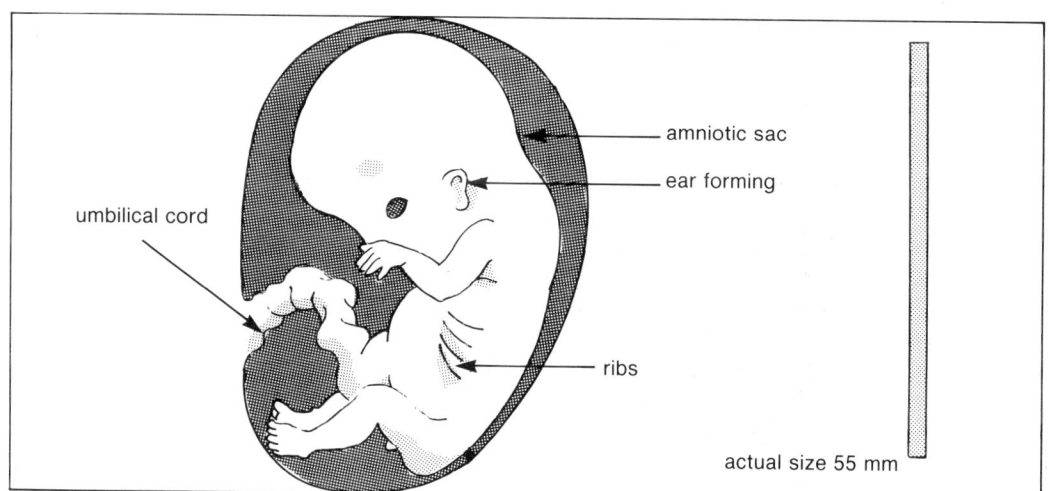

umbilical cord

amniotic sac

ear forming

ribs

actual size 55 mm

The embryo at 10 weeks after conception (12 weeks after the last menstrual period). From now on it becomes a fetus. Its arms and legs have developed fingers and toes, and it looks like a tiny human being

clinic for one or two hours, so that the staff can make sure that the uterus is empty. She may have some crampy pains and, if she has, she will be given analgesic tablets. During the time she is still in the clinic a counsellor will come and talk to her. She will answer any questions the woman may have.

After the operation the woman may bleed for a few days, rather like having a period, or there may be little or no blood lost. The girl returns to the clinic after two weeks to be checked and to talk again about contraception. This reinforces the contraceptive information she was given by her counsellor before she had the abortion.

People may say, 'Abortion sounds so easy, why bother about contraception!' This is foolish. Abortion is not as easy as contraception. It involves an anaesthetic and an operation, and the more abortions a woman has, the greater is the chance of damage to her uterus, so that she is less able to have a baby when she wants one.

The evidence from the USA and Britain is that fewer than 5 per cent of women have a second abortion. Ninety-five per cent of women use contraceptives to prevent another pregnancy.

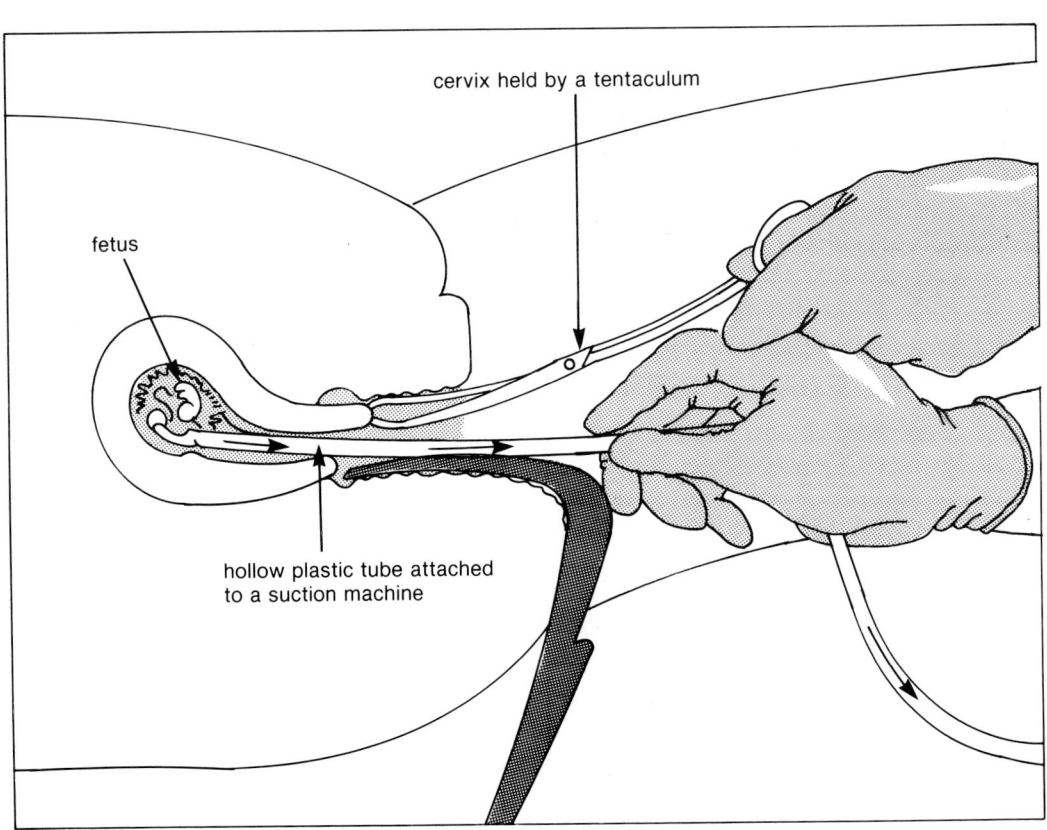

cervix held by a tentaculum

fetus

hollow plastic tube attached to a suction machine

Abortion by suction curettage

*Investigations*

● What are the laws relating to abortion in your State? Are they different in other Australian States?

● Find out all you can about the Menhennit ruling. How did this affect abortion laws?

*Discussions*

● Discuss the effects some abortion pressure groups (for or against) have had on:

(a)  the laws relating to abortion;

(b)  community attitudes to abortion;

(c)  the number of abortions performed.

● Do you think a woman has the right to abortion on demand?

● List some of the reasons a woman might have for seeking an abortion, and discuss the possible consequences of continuing with a pregnancy in the light of these reasons.

# 8

# PREGNANCY AND BIRTH

Pregnancy begins like this. About halfway between a woman's menstrual periods, an ovum is released from her ovary. It comes from the fastest growing of the twenty egg follicles which were stimulated to grow by gonadotrophin hormones during that menstrual cycle.

Shortly after this the follicle bursts and the tiny ovum is set free. It is immediately surrounded by the finger-like fronds at the end of the oviduct and guided inside its tube. If a woman who is not protected against pregnancy has sexual intercourse about the time of ovulation, she will probably become pregnant.

During sexual intercourse the man ejaculates several hundred million sperms into the upper part of the woman's vagina. Of the several hundred million thrashing sperms, only a few hundred thousand manage to navigate through the twisting tunnels which have formed in the mucus of her cervical canal. Several hundred thousand reach the cavity of the uterus but only a few thousand survive to enter the oviducts.

Even then their death-rate is immense. Only a few tens reach the ovum, and only one manages to penetrate its soft 'shell'. Compared with the sperm, the ovum is large. It needs to be because, if pregnancy occurs, it has to supply food for the new being for four days until it is able to obtain its own supply in the uterus.

Within twelve hours of fusion, the fused nuclei divide into two, then divide again into four and again into eight. A new biological life has begun.

For three days the egg is moved towards the uterus by the tiny hairs on many of the cells which line the inner surface of the oviduct. As it moves down its cells continue to divide, so that by the time it enters the uterus on the fourth day it looks like a tiny blackberry. The next day a cavity forms in the 'blackberry', but the egg is still inside the 'shell'. Then, on the fifth day after fertilization, it sheds the 'shell', it fixes itself onto the lining of the uterus, and burrows its way in. It has implanted.

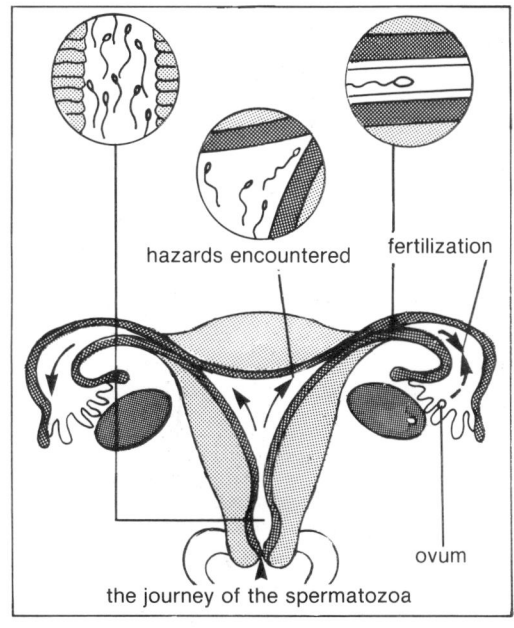

hazards encountered  fertilization

the journey of the spermatozoa

ovum

The development of the ovum, its expulsion from the ovary, and the journey of the sperm

# The first quarter of pregnancy

Only when the ovum has implanted into the uterine lining does it begin to grow in size. The part of the ovum which first attached itself to the uterine lining will become the **placenta**, the rest will form the **embryo**.

The placenta is an organ which provides food for the growing baby. Its cells penetrate the blood vessels which supply the lining of the inside of the uterus and from these it obtains nourishment and oxygen for the baby.

All this happens before the woman has missed a period. By the time her period is due, the placenta is making hormones

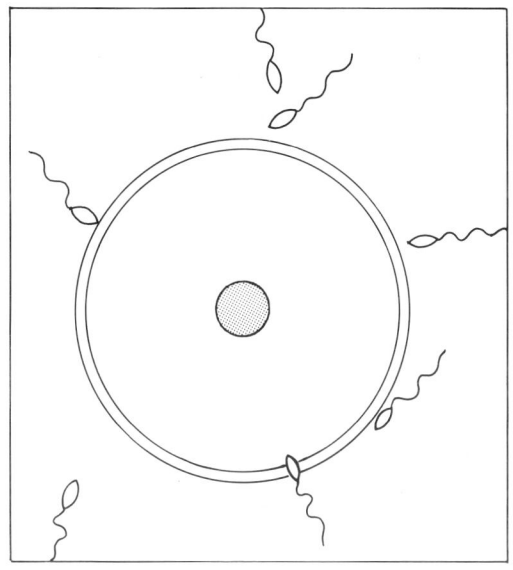

The relative sizes of the sperm and the ovum

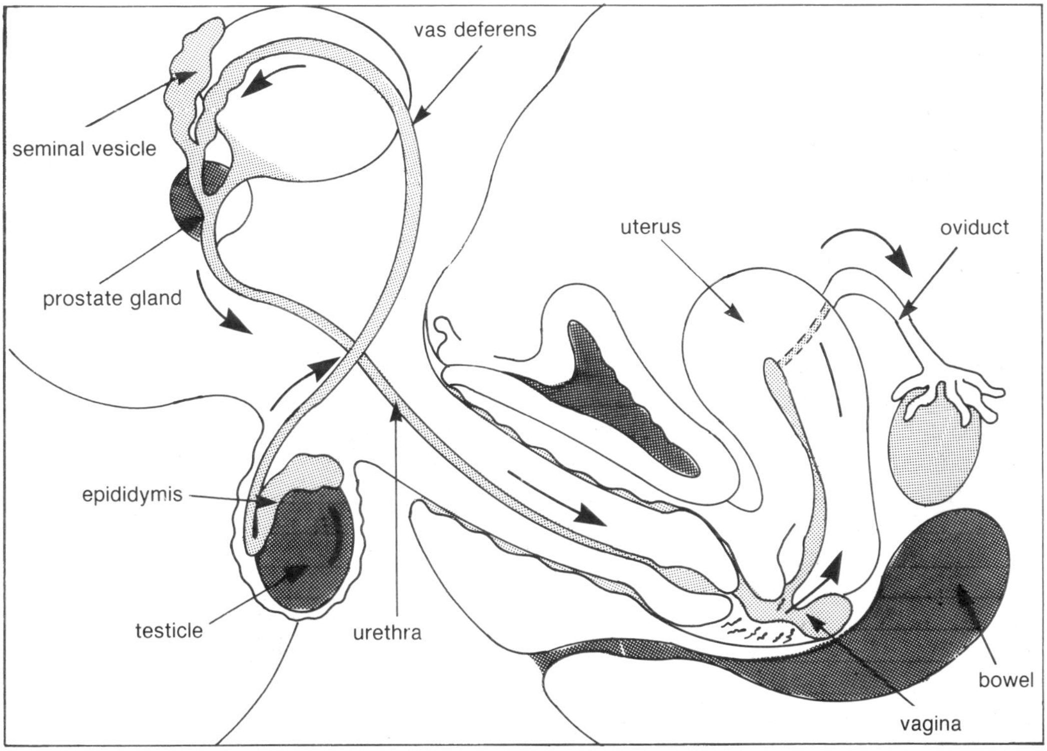

The journey of the spermatozoa

which send messages to the pituitary gland in the brain and to the ovary. These messages stop menstruation occurring.

Once the cells which will form the placenta have fixed firmly to the lining of the uterus, the embryo begins to grow. It looks nothing at all like a human being at this stage. There is a further complication when we talk or write about the embryo. Most people calculate their pregnancy from the first day of the last period, which is convenient but not quite correct. When they say 'I'm eight weeks pregnant', they mean that eight weeks have passed since the first day of the last period. The pregnancy is in fact only six weeks advanced. This confuses people, particularly when they read about an embryo or **fetus** being such and such an age. In this book, each time there is a photograph or a drawing of an embryo or of a fetus, both dates will be shown on the caption.

By the sixth week from the last period, the fourth week in the life of the embryo, it is still unrecognizable as a human being. It looks a little like a tiny reptile as it floats inside a small sac it has made to protect itself. It is only about 5 mm long.

The woman is now two weeks past her expected period and wonders if she could be pregnant. She can find out by having a pregnancy test done. The test depends on the presence of a special pregnancy hormone, made by the placenta, in the woman's blood or urine. A test which is positive for the hormone, called human

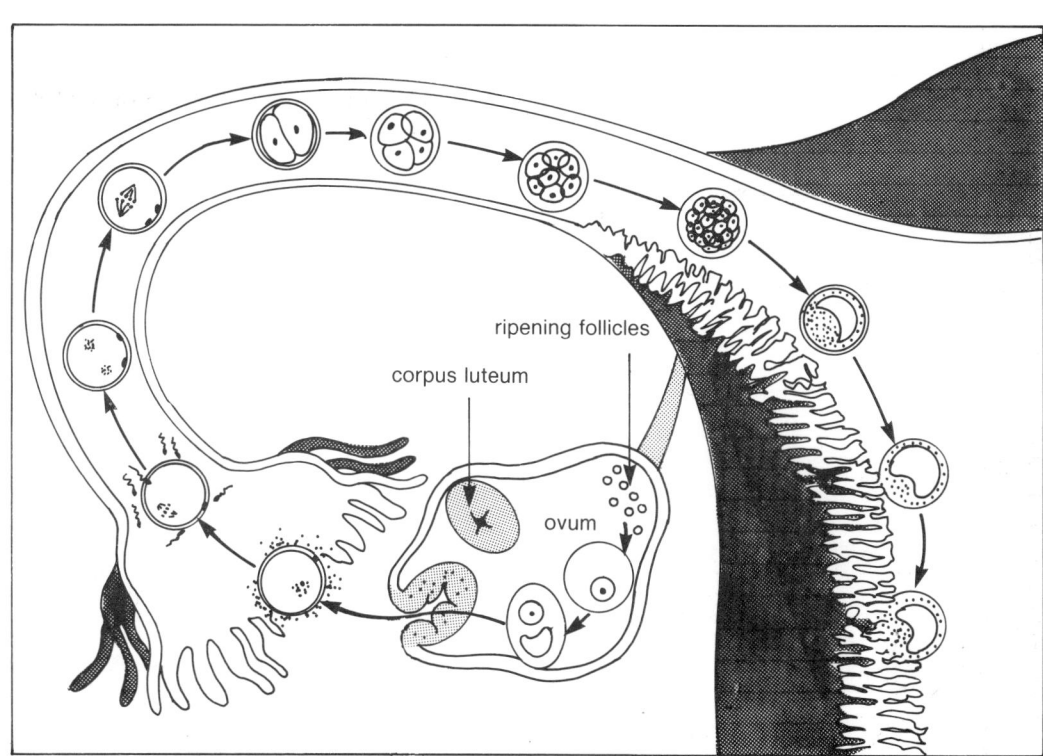

The beginning of pregnancy. The development of the embryo from fertilization until it is fixed to the wall of the uterus takes about four days

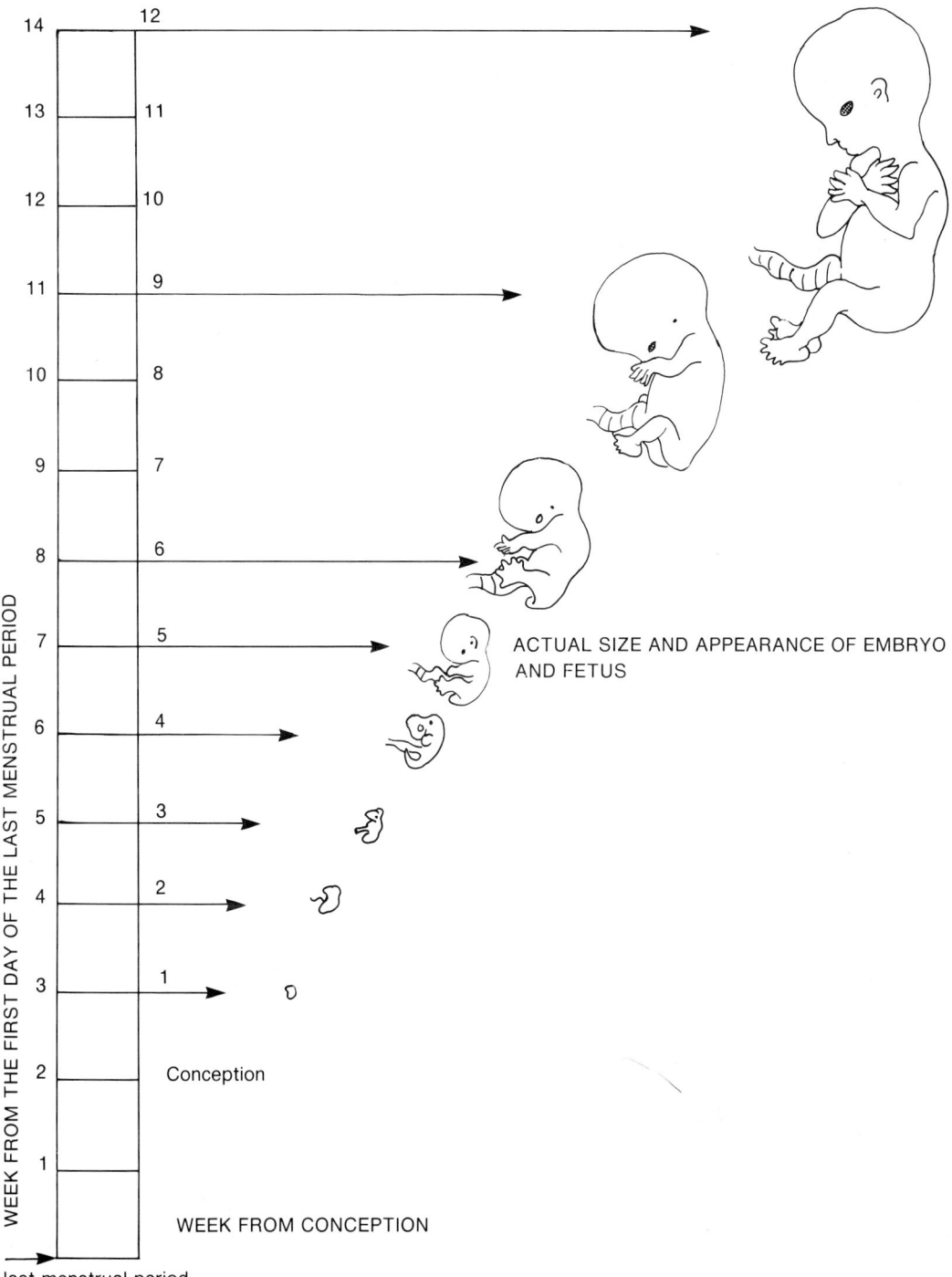

WEEK FROM THE FIRST DAY OF THE LAST MENSTRUAL PERIOD

14 — 12

13 — 11

12 — 10

11 — 9

10 — 8

9 — 7

8 — 6

7 — 5

6 — 4

5 — 3

4 — 2

3 — 1

2    Conception

1

WEEK FROM CONCEPTION

last menstrual period

ACTUAL SIZE AND APPEARANCE OF EMBRYO AND FETUS

**chronic gonadotrophin**, indicates that the woman is pregnant. Recently a new pregnancy test, using a technique called monoclonal antibodies, enables a woman to tell if she is pregnant within six days of the date of her missed period.

Around the time of her second missed period the woman may begin to feel a little nauseated, especially in the morning; and her breasts may be getting heavier. By now the embryo is six weeks old. It is about 10 mm long and has begun to resemble a human—a very primitive human. It has a big irregular shaped head and two blind eyes. It has started growing buds at the end of its limbs, which will turn into hands and feet. At the moment there is just a suggestion of fingers and toes. By the end of the tenth week from the last menstrual period a woman can be sure she is pregnant. Her doctor, examining her internally, can tell that the uterus is enlarged and soft. She feels pregnant. The embryo, now about 30–40 mm long, is eight weeks old. It looks much more like a human. Its heart has been beating for about four weeks and its eyes appear to be open because it has no eyelids. One-quarter of the pregnancy has passed.

All the organs which make up a human body have been formed. Although they will go through many changes in shape and size before the baby is born, this is the end of organ formation (called **embryogenesis**). From this time on the embryo, now just recognizable as a human, is called a fetus.

By the end of the twelfth week after the start of the last menstruation, the fetus is ten weeks old. It looks human, and is nearly 40–50 mm long. It has proper arms and legs which it moves regularly. Its head is now more in proportion to its body. It has a large forehead and a definite chin. Its forehead wrinkles, its lips open and close, but it is still tiny, weighing only 20 g. It is protected from injury, from changes of temperature, and is able to move about, because it is in a water-filled bag called the **amniotic sac**. It is connected to the placenta by the **umbilical cord** alone.

The fetus can be compared with an astronaut in a space capsule, floating about, almost weightless, in a heat-controlled, oxygen-controlled space, connected to its support system (the placenta) by a tube (the umbilical cord).

# Spontaneous abortion (miscarriage)

Not all babies develop in this way. In about one pregnancy in every ten the fetus doesn't form properly, and a spontaneous abortion or miscarriage occurs. The fetus may hardly form at all, or it may form and then die. Its support system, the placenta, also functions poorly, and its special hormones cease to be made. This means that the uterus no longer accepts the improperly formed fetus and tries to expel it. The woman begins to bleed from her uterus and may have crampy pains.

The doctor may be able to tell whether a woman is going to abort a fetus that hasn't

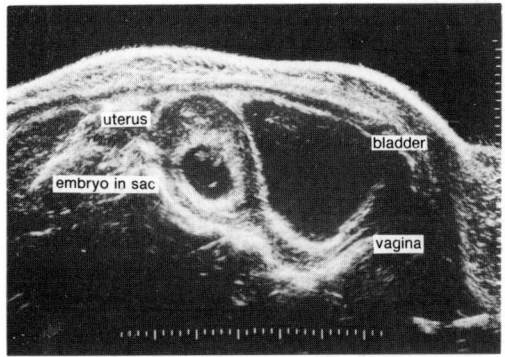

An ultrasound picture of a nine-week-old embryo in its sac inside the uterus

formed properly, or whether everything is normal, by examining her vaginally. Sometimes he is wrong! Today, a machine called an ultrasound machine helps. By using sound waves it can make a picture of the uterus, showing if there is a normal fetus or one which hasn't formed properly. It can also find if the fetus's heart is beating.

If the miscarriage is going to occur, the bleeding usually becomes heavier and the crampy pains stronger. If this happens it is wise to go to hospital so that, if necessary, drugs to reduce the pain can be given, and the uterus can be helped to expel the baby.

# What to do if you are pregnant

Pregnancy in teenagers, especially young teenagers, that is women aged sixteen or less, carries greater risks than pregnancy in women aged from twenty to thirty. The main problems are that more teenaged expectant mothers are anaemic or develop a raised blood pressure in pregnancy. These problems, and others, increase the chance that the birth weight of the baby will be low. In fact, mothers aged nineteen or less are one and a half times more likely to give birth to a low-birth-weight baby than mothers aged between twenty and twenty-nine. Low birth weight increases the chance that the baby will die; and there is a higher perinatal mortality—deaths of babies around the time of birth—among babies born to teenaged mothers.

The main reason for the increase in pregnancy problems and for the low birth weight of the babies seems to be that some teenagers conceal the pregnancy and delay obtaining the ante-natal care which can help to prevent problems developing.

If a teenager suspects that she is pregnant and the pregnancy is unwanted and unwelcome, she should see a doctor two weeks after her first missed period, that is, six weeks after her last menstruation.

At this early stage of pregnancy she may wish to talk to her doctor (or to the social workers who are attached to most hospitals) about her worries and any problems she may have. It may be that she has thought about having an abortion. This can be discussed. It may be that she has decided to continue with the pregnancy. By seeing her doctor at an early stage of pregnancy, she can be examined to confirm that she is physically and emotionally healthy. Blood tests can be made to check her blood group and to make sure that she is not anaemic. The doctor will usually examine her vaginally and will be able to tell her when the baby's birth may be expected.

The social workers can help her to overcome the many problems which may arise if she decides not to marry the baby's father. They are trained to help people and can talk over the anxieties, the fears, and the concerns that many pregnant women have. In recent years most unmarried teenage mothers have chosen to keep and rear their babies, and fewer than 10 per cent of teenage mothers have decided to give their babies away for adoption. The help the social workers can give a teenage mother in learning about the services available to help her during her pregnancy, and afterwards as a single parent, is becoming increasingly important.

The doctor, the nurse, the social worker or the dietitian will also talk with the expectant mother about what she should eat during pregnancy so that her baby obtains the best possible nourishment whilst it is in her uterus. The growth of the baby and its health after it is born depend, to some extent, on what the expectant mother eats during pregnancy. Many teenagers eat 'schluck' food. They eat too many sweet things, too many pre-cooked takeaway foods, and too many soft drinks. A pregnant woman should cut down on sugar, pastries and cakes, and should eat more fresh fruit, vegetables, eggs, milk, and protein in the form of lean meat, chicken or fish. She may be given vitamin pills to supplement her diet, but for most people eating a good diet they are not necessary.

The expectant mother can also ask her doctor questions about things which worry her. Even if the question seems trivial, an expectant mother should ask it—it is important to her or she wouldn't want to ask! She may want to know about sex, but is often embarrassed to ask, and the doctor usually doesn't mention the subject. A woman can be reassured that she can enjoy sex all through pregnancy without any danger of damage to herself or to the baby.

The doctor, or the nurse, will outline for the expectant mother how often she should visit the surgery or the clinic during pregnancy and what tests will be made. Her blood will be re-tested at the beginning of the fourth quarter of pregnancy (about the thirtieth week from the date of her last

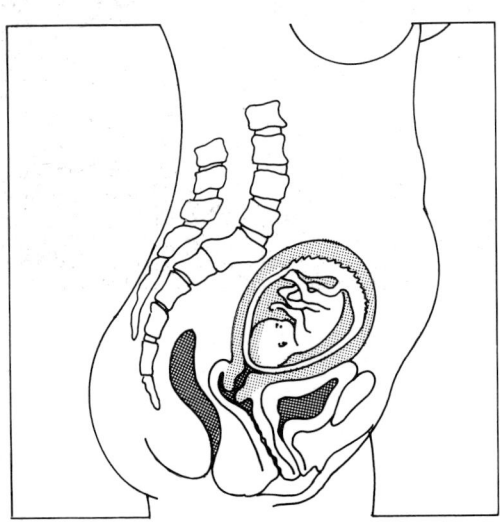

Fetus at sixteen weeks since the last menstrual period (fourteen weeks since conception)

menstrual period). The doctor will expect her to visit every month until she is twenty-eight weeks pregnant, then every two weeks until she is thirty-six weeks pregnant, and then every week until the baby is born.

These visits are for the purpose of checking the expectant mother and her baby, to see how both are enjoying the pregnancy.

At the check-up in the sixteenth week, the bulge in the woman's belly is beginning to be visible. The baby (now fourteen weeks old) is about 160–180 mm long and weighs about 100 g. Its sex can now be distinguished easily. The mother begins to feel the fetus moving. This is called 'quickening', because at one time it was believed that only at this time did the baby become alive or 'quick'.

# The second half of pregnancy

At the check-up in the twentieth week the woman is half-way through the pregnancy. Her uterus now reaches her umbilicus and is stretching her abdomen. The baby is now eighteen weeks old, about 200–250 mm long, and it weighs about 400 g. Its eyes are closed, as its eyelids have now formed. Its body is covered with fine hair, called **lanugo**. It can suck its fingers. If it is born now, it has a faint chance of surviving —with good luck and good care.

Four weeks later, at the check-up in the twenty-four week, the baby has grown to be about 300–350 mm long and it weighs 650 g. Its skin is less red because it is beginning to make a protective greasy substance called **vernix**. It is wrinkled because it has very little fat beneath its skin. Its lungs are still very immature so that if it is born now it may have great difficulty in breathing.

By the twenty-eighth week of preg-

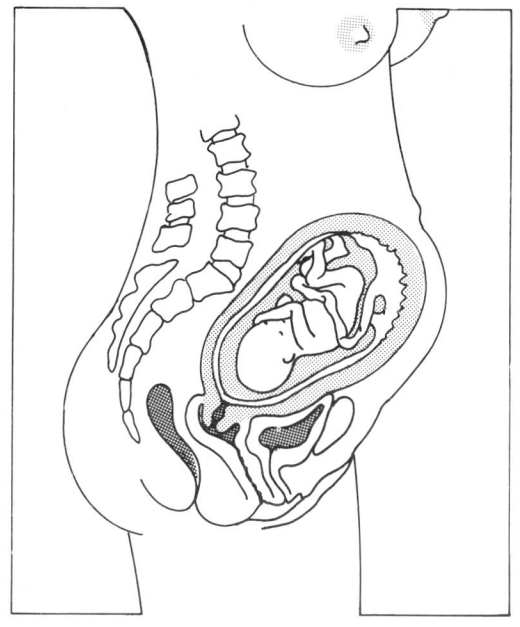

Fetus at twenty weeks since the last menstrual period (eighteen weeks since conception)

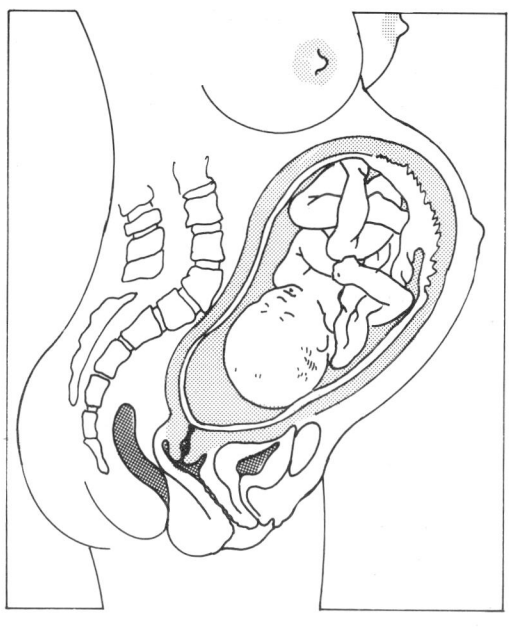

Fetus at thirty-two weeks since the last menstrual period (thirty weeks since conception)

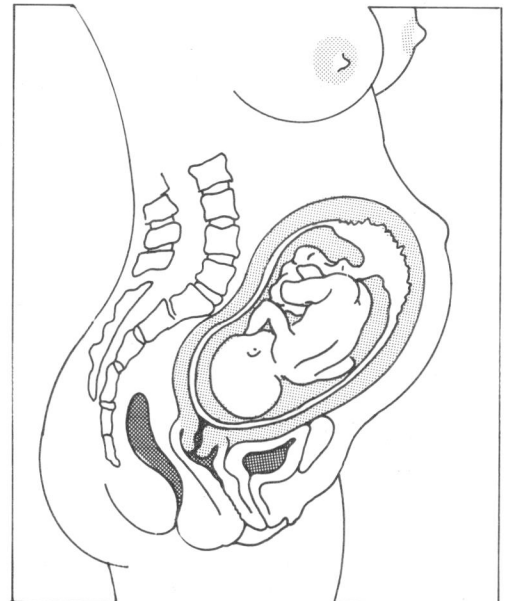

Fetus at twenty-four weeks since the last menstrual period (twenty-two weeks since conception)

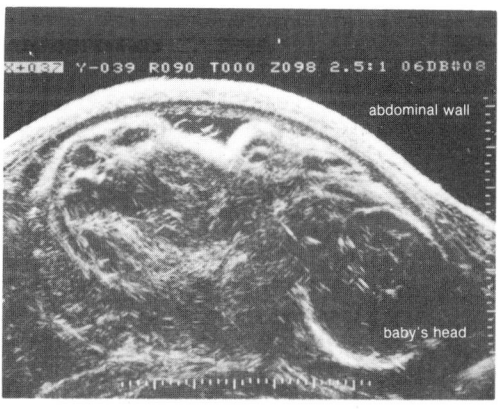

An ultrasound picture of a fetus at thirty-six weeks since the last menstrual period (thirty-four weeks since conception)

nancy, the baby is about 350–400 mm long and weighs about 1000 g. It can now open its eyes, and if it is born can breathe, although it may need help. It has a 70 per cent chance of surviving outside the womb if it is treated in a special unit for small babies.

At the end of the thirty-second week, the expectant mother has a large bulge in her abdomen. The baby is now about 450 mm long and weighs about 1800 g. Eight out of every ten babies born at this stage will survive.

By the thirty-sixth week the mother is getting close to the date of her baby's birth. Her uterus reaches all the way up to her rib cage. To keep her balance she has to push her shoulders back. Varicose veins in the legs can become a problem at this stage of pregnancy. The baby is now about 450–500 mm long and weighs about 2500 g. It has gained nearly 750 g in the last four weeks because it now has fat beneath its skin. Its body is rounded. If it is born now, it has a 95 per cent chance of surviving.

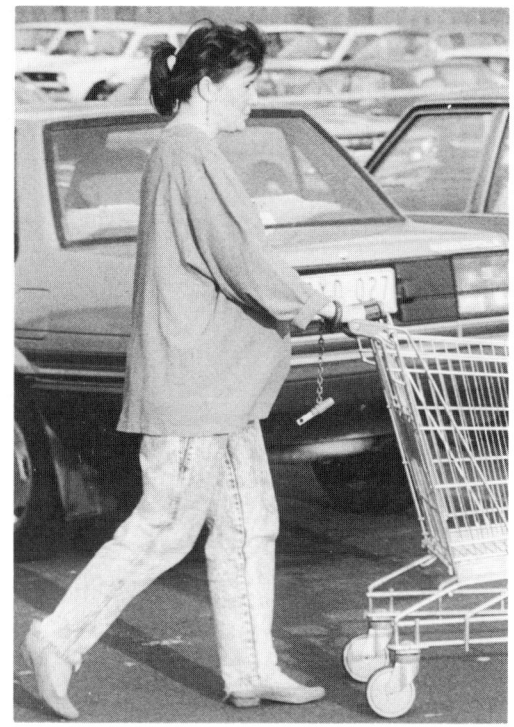

# Why an expectant mother should go to the clinic regularly

The visits to the doctor or the clinic have several purposes. The doctor can check that the expectant mother is well and, particularly, that her blood pressure has not risen. Teenaged expectant mothers are rather more likely than older women to develop a raised blood pressure in the second half of pregnancy; about one in ten does. The raised blood pressure may get worse and may threaten the life of the baby or, although rarely today, the mother's life. The condition is called toxaemia or, more correctly, pregnancy-induced hypertension.

At each visit the doctor will also check that the baby is growing properly and what its position is inside the uterus. If the doctor is in any doubt about the baby's health, tests on the expectant mother's urine or her blood may be made. If the doctor is in doubt about the baby's position or whether it is growing properly, an ultrasound picture will be taken.

Most babies lie head down by the thirty-sixth week of pregnancy. Soon after this date, the lower part of the uterus stretches and the head drops to fit snugly into the bones of its mother's pelvis. It is getting ready to be born.

# Childbirth or labour

The expected date of the baby's birth, which the expectant mother was given at the first visit to the doctor, is an average

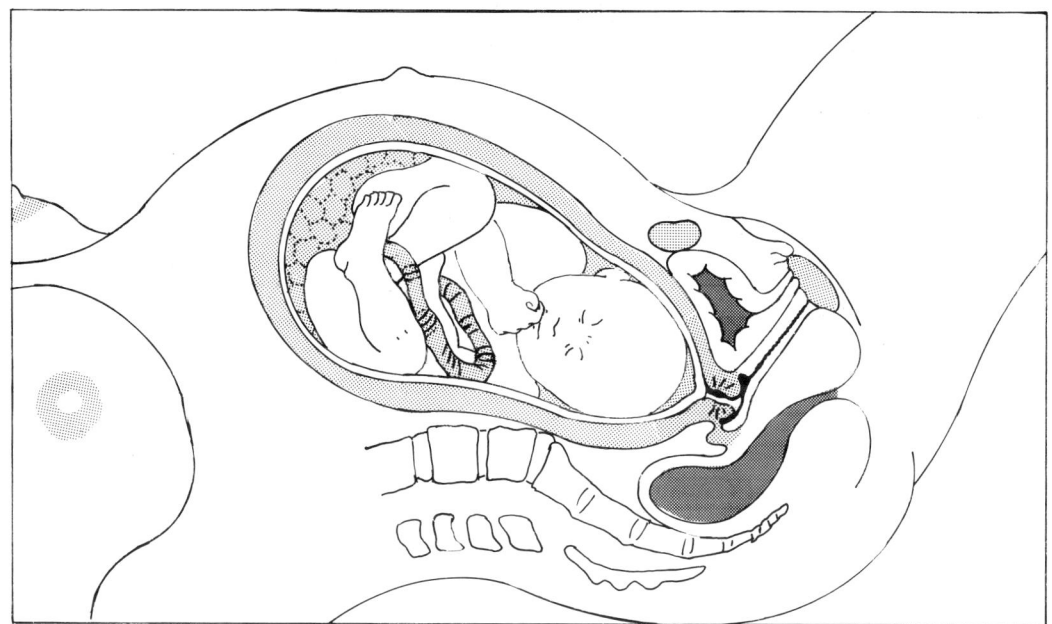

The baby in late pregnancy. Its head has settled
into the mother's pelvis. The cervix is soft but has
not yet been drawn up

date. Humans vary and it is quite normal for the baby to be born two weeks before or two weeks after the expected date.

We don't know why a woman starts in labour when she does. In spite of much research, the reasons are still a mystery.

By the time her baby is due to be born the mother may have been feeling some discomfort in her pelvis for two or three weeks, and she may have noticed that her uterus was contracting quite strongly from time to time. These practice contractions are known as Braxton-Hicks contractions.

When the baby is ready to be born the contractions become regular in duration and intervals between them decrease. The mother may notice a sticky blood-stained discharge coming from her vagina; this is called a 'show', and is caused by the cervix of the uterus starting to open.

In childbirth several things happen. During the first stage of labour, the cervix has to open progressively until it is fully open and the cavity of the uterus and that of the vagina make a single tube. This takes on average about eight to nine hours, but can take a shorter or a longer time.

The cervix is opened by the contractions of the uterus, which get stronger and more intense as labour progresses. These contractions are experienced by the mother as wavelike, often very intense, sensations. Then, usually when the cervix is fully open, the amniotic sac (bag of water), which has protected the baby through pregnancy, breaks. A gush of water floods through the vagina and the baby's head presses in the pelvis. The second stage of labour, when the mother can help to give birth to her baby, has begun.

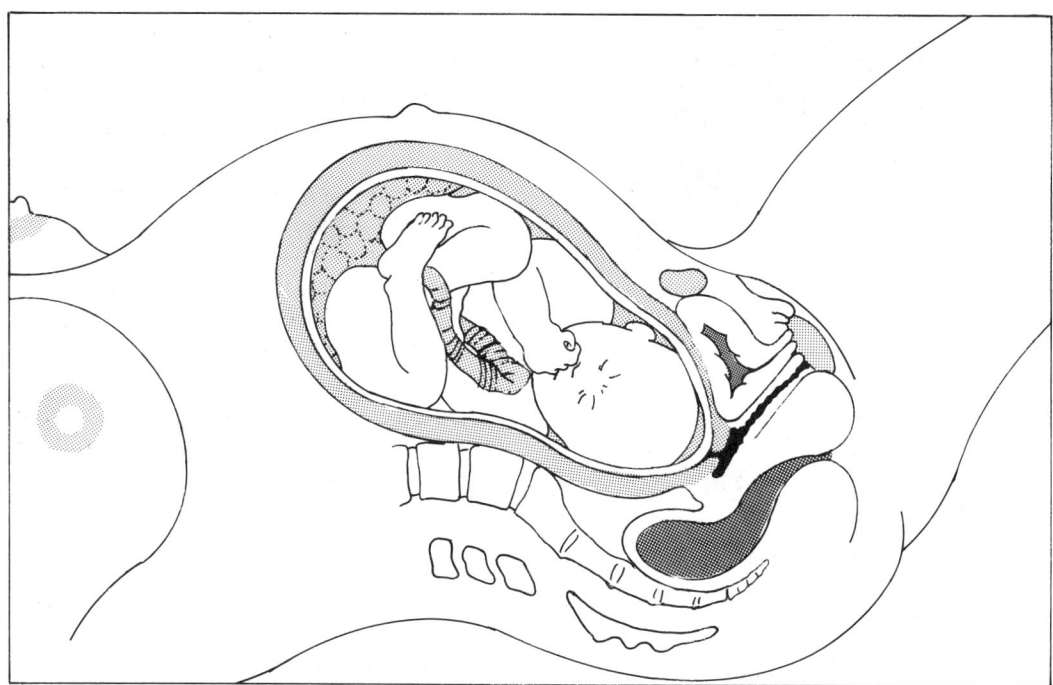

The position of the baby in early labour

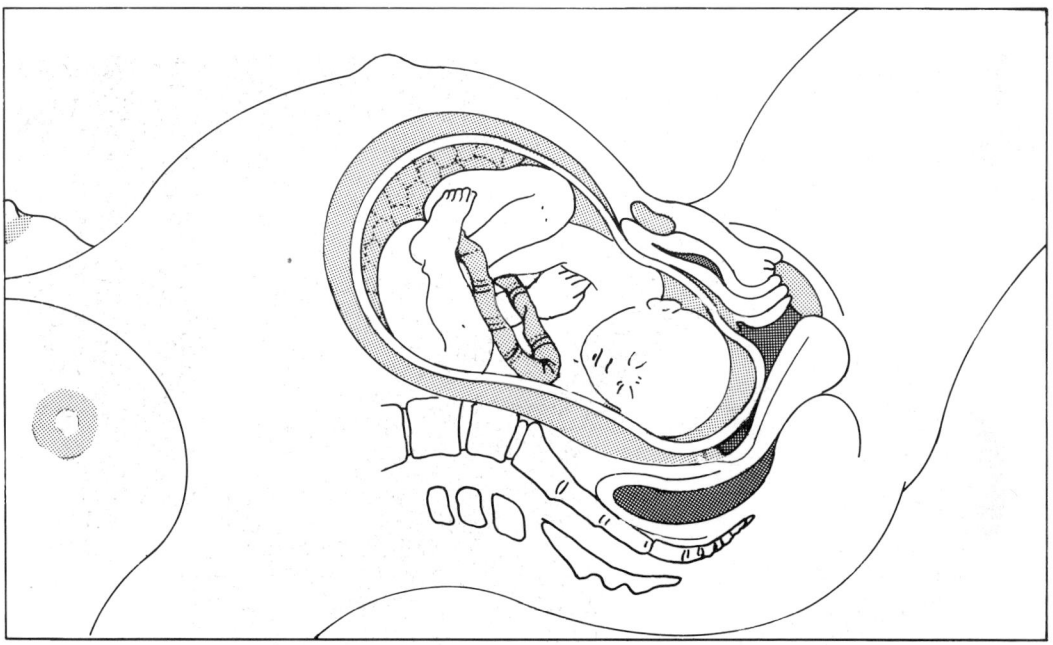

The cervix has almost completely opened by the
end of the first stage of labour

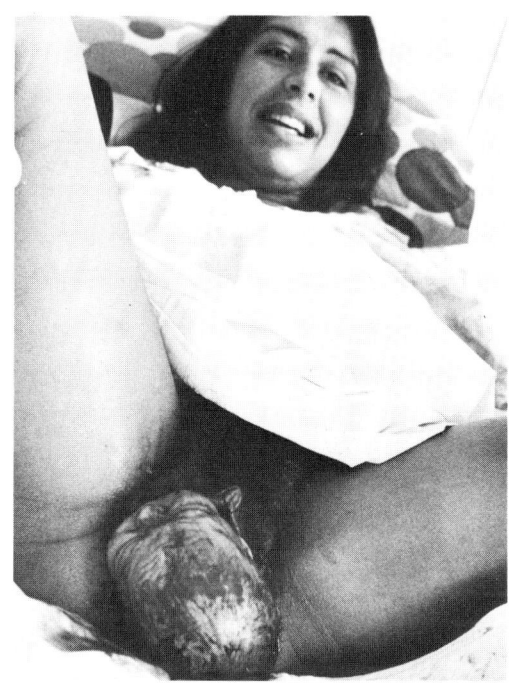

Now each contraction pushes the baby further down the vagina, or birth canal. The mother can help by contracting her abdominal muscles and her diaphragm and pushing.

In about twenty to forty minutes—though in some cases it takes less and in some more time—the baby's head is visible at the vulva, and within about twenty minutes (though again this is only an average time; the actual time can vary) the baby is born.

It lies stretching and often crying between its mother's legs. The umbilical cord ceases to beat and is cut, and the mother may have her baby to caress, talk to and suckle.

A few minutes later (in most cases) the placenta ('after-birth') is expelled from the uterus. If the mother needs stitches because of a tear in the perineum (see p. 9) caused by the birth of the baby, the doctor puts these in.

The baby's head is born

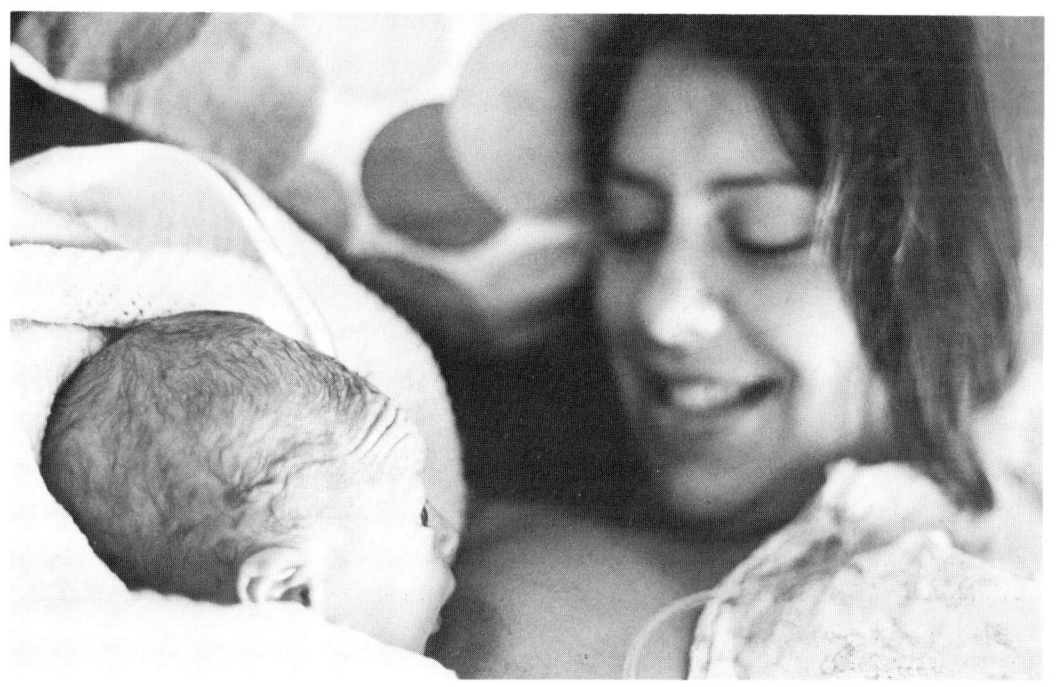

# Choices in childbirth

Women and their partners have a choice to make. They have to decide how they want to have their baby born.

They can choose to have as 'natural' a childbirth as possible. This means that, in hospital births, the room in the hospital is made as much like a bedroom as possible. The father of the baby, and perhaps some relative or friend chosen by the expectant mother, stays with her, supporting and helping her. She is only given drugs if and when she asks for them. The birth of the baby is gentle and quiet, without bright lights. The newborn baby is given at once to the mother to hold, to caress and to suckle. From this time on the baby stays with the mother in her room. For this method to succeed, both parents need to learn about the process of childbirth and parenting. It helps them if they go to classes so that they are prepared for child-birth.

This means that both have a clear mental picture of what is happening during the birth of their child, and that they have learnt simple breathing techniques which will enable the woman to relax during the contractions of the first stage of labour and to help push out the baby in the second stage. For prepared childbirth to work there has to be maturity and self-confidence, and some degree of loving co-operation between the participants.

The expectant parents may not wish to have this kind of childbirth. In many cultures, childbirth is a matter for women only. The expectant father doesn't want to be involved until the baby is born, when he expects to be congratulated by all the neighbours. In this method in developed countries, the expectant mother goes into hospital when she thinks that labour has started. She is looked after by the nurses in a 'delivery room', which is full of equipment and brightly lit. She is given pain-relieving injections when she thinks she needs them. She gives birth to the baby, and after holding it for a while, it is taken away to be weighed and washed before being returned to her. In the next few days the baby spends some time with her, but for some of the time it lives in a nursery, with all the other babies.

The third choice is to have a 'technological' birth. The expectant mother and the doctor agree on what day the baby will be born. Early that morning the doctor examines the woman internally to check that the baby is ready to be born. If it is, he ruptures the amniotic sac by inserting a small instrument through the woman's cervix, and the 'waters' gush out. He sets up a drip into a vein in the woman's arm and through it gives a substance, called oxytocin, which makes the uterus contract.

Because labour has been started 'artificially' he attaches a machine called a cardiotocograph to the woman. This monitors the contractions of the uterus and the baby's heart rate so that abnormalities in either can be detected early. The contractions tend to become strong and painful quickly. To relieve the pain an anaesthetist gives an injection called an epidural into the woman's spine. This stops all the pain, but permits the contractions to continue. When the baby's head is visible at the vulva, the doctor makes a small cut in the skin of the perineum and usually delivers the baby with forceps.

Women should have the right to choose which method suits them best. However, if the baby is at special risk, the doctor may have to decide on a particular method, usually a modification of 'technological' childbirth, because it is safer for both the baby and the mother. This decision only has to be made in about fifteen per cent of labours—most labours proceed normally, and safely.

Whichever method of childbirth is chosen by the mother and her partner, it is important that the baby be born in a place where urgent action can be taken should an emergency arise. In most places in Australia today, this means that the safest place for having babies is a hospital. A home birth is only a responsible alternative if a qualified, trained and experienced midwife or a doctor is present. The mother should have been cared for by the midwife or the doctor throughout her pregnancy.

## Parenting

The birth of the baby is the beginning of being a parent. Parenting is not instinctive; it has to be learned.

We know that it is important for the baby and the mother to be left together for as much time as possible immediately after the birth and during the first days of the baby's life. This leads to a close bond between mother and baby. Early contact between the father and the baby helps the development of a close relationship between them also. This early bonding helps the parenting process. We know too that it is important for a mother to breast feed her baby if she can. Over 95 per cent of mothers are able to breast feed if they learn about breast feeding during pregnancy, prepare their nipples, and are helped to establish breast feeding after birth (the Nursing Mothers' Association of Australia provides information and counselling about breast feeding). Breast feeding is important as it also creates a close and loving link between the mother and her baby. Human milk is better for the baby than cow's milk (however much this is modified in formula baby milks which you

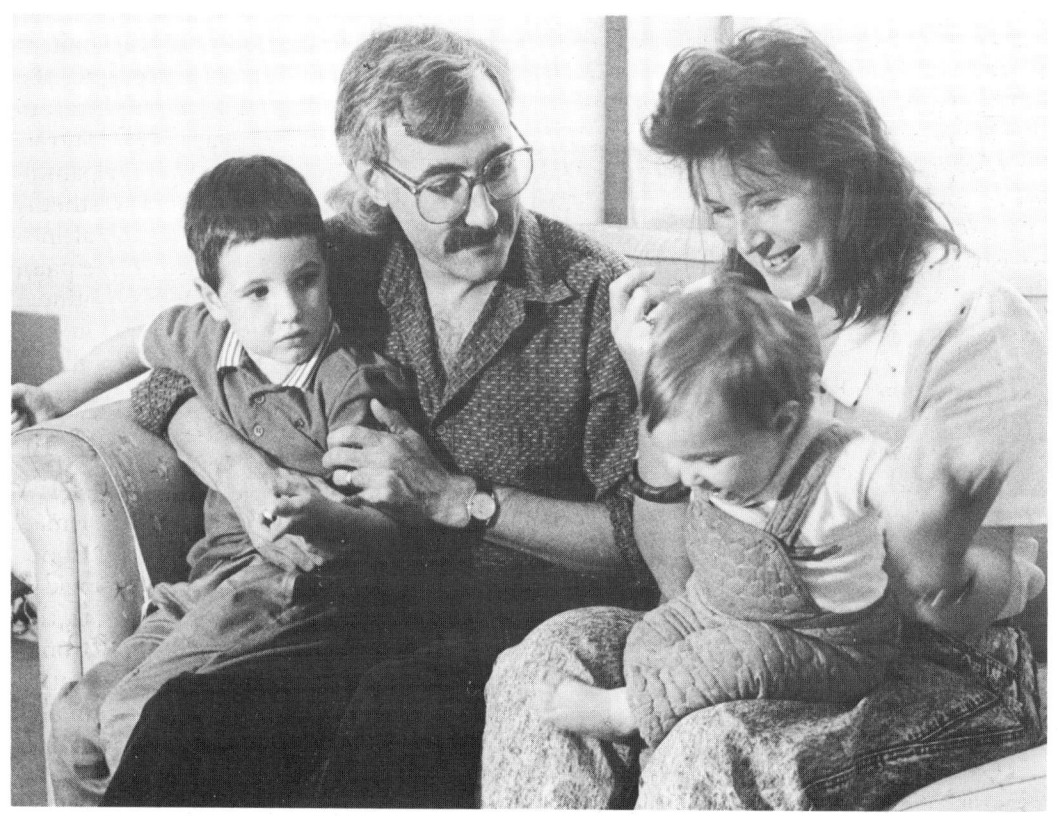

buy from the supermarket or chemist). Human milk protects the baby against many infections. Breast fed babies are less likely to become fat, and to develop milk allergies. Breast feeding is more convenient and costs less than bottle feeding.

We now know that it is important for both parents to help care for the baby. This helps to reduce the strain on the mother of having to look after a baby, a husband and a home, and it increases a bond between father and child. This is especially important today, as other relatives who might help, such as mother or mother-in-law, aunts or sisters-in-law, are often too busy or live too far away.

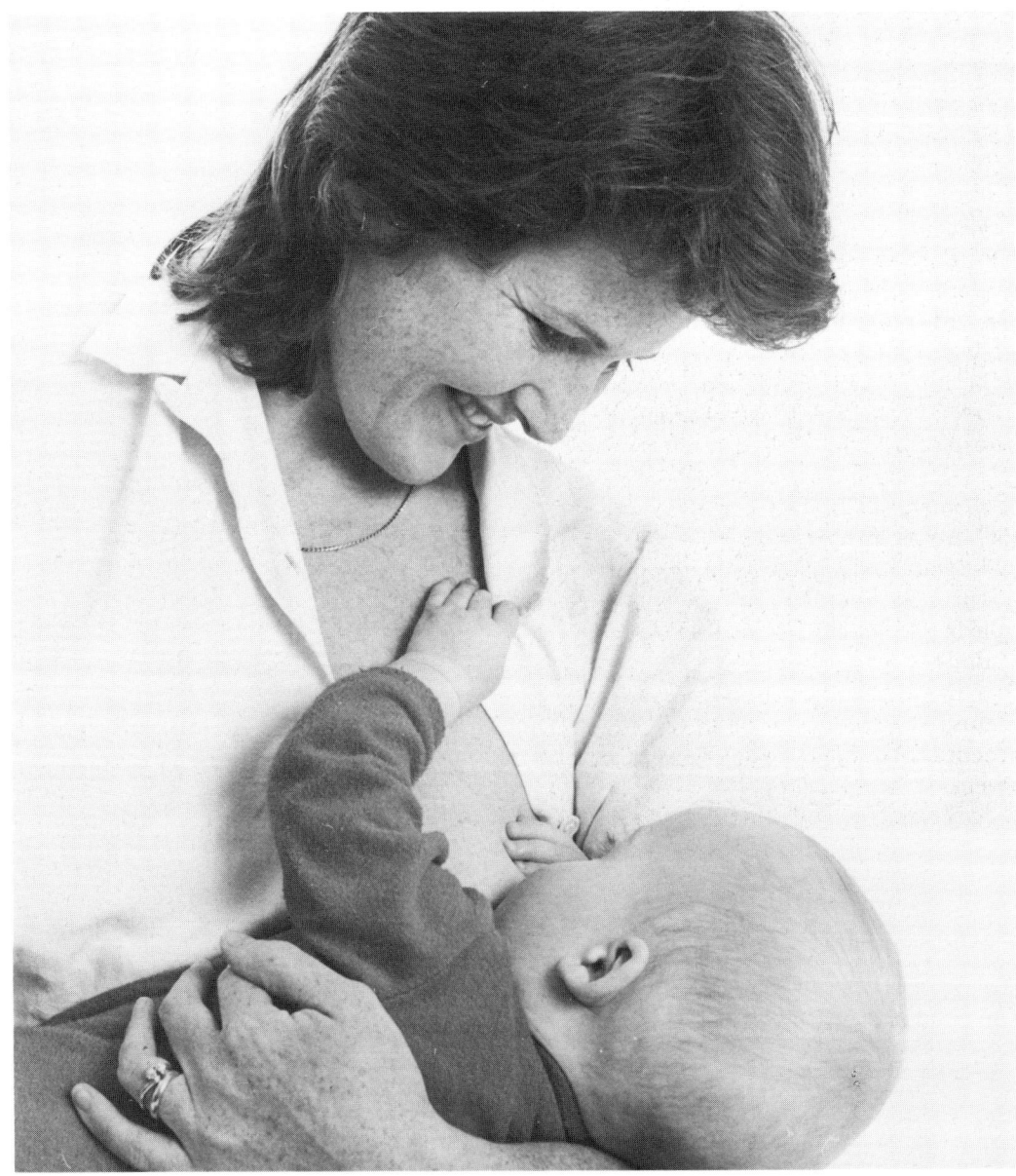

*Investigations*
- Find out about customs related to pregnancy and childbirth in other cultures.
- Find out all you can about the Leboyer method of childbirth.
- Investigate the possible effects on the fetus of a mother's
(a) smoking;
(b) taking pain-killing drugs;
(c) taking any other kind of drugs;
(d) diet;
(e) exercise;
(f) thoughts and feelings.

*Discussions*
- Describe the birth of a child from the point of view of a spectator.
- What are your feelings about the advantages and disadvantages of home and hospital births? Talk to people who have experienced births at home and in hospitals.

*Activities*
- Arrange to have a speaker from the Childbirth Education Association talk to your class about pregnancy and child-birth and how they involve the whole family.
- Draw or make life-size models of the fetus at the various stages of development: six weeks, twelve weeks, sixteen weeks, twenty weeks.

# 9

# THE INFERTILE COUPLE

When a couple decides to have a baby, most find that they achieve the pregnancy within one year of trying.

However, some can't. About one couple in every ten fails to achieve the desired pregnancy.

This can cause them much distress, and it is usual, in our culture, for the wife to be the first to consult a doctor because of infertility.

## The causes of infertility

Infertility has many causes, but certain broad problems can be outlined once you know what to look for.

As we discussed in the last chapter, for a pregnancy to occur:
● The woman has to develop and then expel an ovum from one of her ovaries.
● The ovum has to enter the oviduct.
● Within two days before or after ovulation, the man has to ejaculate a large number of good quality sperm in the woman's vagina.
● Millions of these sperm have to wriggle and twist through the secretions of the cervix of the uterus.
● Hundreds have to survive the journey through the cavity of the uterus.
● Tens have to get into the opening of the oviduct and swim along it, against the current.

● A single sperm has to penetrate the 'shell' of the ovum and its head has to fuse with the nucleus in the ovum.
● The new being has to form properly, dividing repeatedly in the five days it takes for the fertilized egg to reach the cavity of the uterus.
● The fertilized egg has to implant in the lining of the uterus and grow.

Anything which prevents this sequence of events will prevent or will hinder pregnancy.

## The man

In over one-third of cases of infertility, the man is the problem. In most cases he is able to get an erection and to enjoy sexual intercourse, but when he ejaculates he spurts either few or no sperm from his penis. A man can be tested to find out the quality and the quantity of his sperm quite easily. He masturbates, and ejaculates into a clean dry jar. The jar containing semen is taken to a laboratory and examined.

If the quality of his semen is normal, he is not the cause of the problem. But if his semen is of poor quality, or if no sperm are found in it, the test is repeated and a blood test is made. Unfortunately, there isn't anything that can be done if he has no sperm. In a few cases only can poor quality semen be improved.

## The woman

The woman checks if she is ovulating by taking her temperature each morning. It has been found that after ovulation the body temperature rises slightly. Blood tests can also be made to confirm ovulation.

The doctor needs to find out if the oviducts are open so that the sperm can swim along them to reach the ovum, and so that the fertilized ovum can be moved gently along the oviduct to reach the uterus. The doctor tests this in two ways. First, a narrow tube can be put into the cervix and attached to a syringe. A substance which is visible on X-ray is injected, and the uterus and oviducts are outlined. If the oviducts are open the substance escapes into the abdominal cavity. The other way the doctor can do the test is to make a small cut in a woman's umbilicus and put a narrow telescope-like instrument, called a laparoscope, into her abdomen. He then injects a blue dye into the uterus. Looking through the laparoscope he can observe if the dye appears. If the oviducts are blocked no dye will be seen. If the woman has blocked oviducts she can't get pregnant. Occasionally, surgery is used to cut out the block and rejoin the good parts of the oviducts. Unfortunately the success rate, judged by

whether the woman is then able to conceive and give birth to a live baby, is less than 20 per cent.

A few infertile women either do not ovulate at all or only ovulate irregularly. These women can now be helped to conceive by taking one of the fertility pills or injections. But these women account for only a very few infertility problems.

Other tests are also sometimes made, particularly to see if the sperm can wriggle through the cervical secretions or not, but they have not been proved to help much in increasing the number of pregnancies.

# What can be done?

The tests, which may themselves be a form of treatment, and the few specific treatments doctors can give, enable about 45 per cent of infertile couples to have a pregnancy within one year, and a few more in the next three or four years.

## Artificial insemination

If the man has no sperm, nothing can be done to help the couple achieve a pregnancy. They can decide to adopt a baby, or

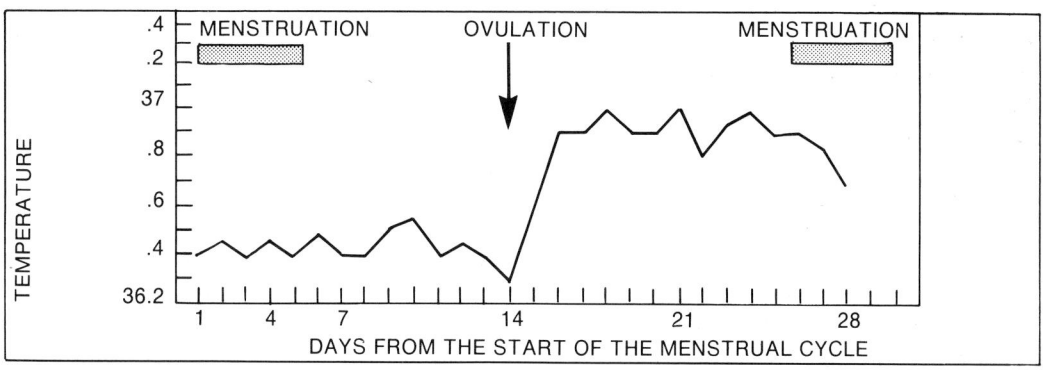

A temperature chart showing that ovulation has occurred on day 14

they may choose for the wife to try to have a baby following an injection into her cervix of the semen of a fertile man. This is called AID—artificial insemination by a donor.

The actual procedure is simple. The woman is taught to work out when she is ovulating. On that day she goes to a special clinic where she will have to stay for about an hour. The clinic either has frozen sperm available or else gets a donor to provide fresh sperm by masturbating. The sperm is injected into her cervix on that day, and the procedure is repeated on the next day.

The organization for an AID service is more complicated. Neither husband nor wife must know who the donor is, nor must the donor know to whom his sperm has been given. The donor must be healthy and have been checked for various diseases, including AIDS. More pregnancies are said to occur if fresh semen is injected, but this requires more organization. If frozen sperm is used it has to be collected, checked, and snap-frozen using liquid nitrogen.

If AID is used for three successive months at ovulation time, about half the women inseminated will have become pregnant—which is not a bad result for a complicated procedure. If AID is continued for a further six months a few more women become pregnant.

## In-vitro fertilization

Women whose oviducts are irreparably damaged or blocked had no chance until recently of becoming pregnant. Now they have a twenty per cent chance. This is due to the development of in-vitro fertilization. At the time of ovulation an egg (ovum) is removed from the woman's ovary by introducing a narrow tube into her abdomen. The egg is placed in a test-tube in a nutrient broth and about five hours later her partner's sperm is added after special treat-

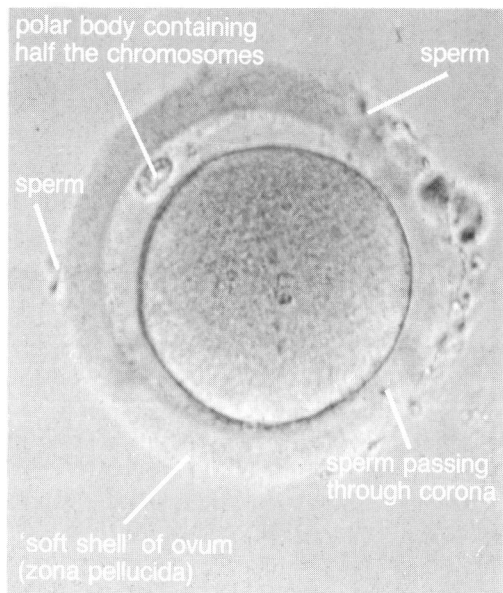

polar body containing half the chromosomes

sperm

sperm

sperm passing through corona

'soft shell' of ovum (zona pellucida)

In-vitro fertilization

1

ment. The test-tube is examined under a microscope to see if the egg is fertilized. About forty hours later, the fertilized egg (now an embryo) is sucked into a tube attached to a small syringe. The tube is introduced into the uterus through the cervix. The embryo is gently injected into the cavity of the uterus. It has been replaced into its mother's womb.

Recent developments in in-vitro fertilization include inducing multiple ovulation (by using fertility pills) and then fertilizing several eggs to produce several embryos. Two or three embryos are introduced into the mother's uterus and the rest are frozen in liquid nitrogen. If the embryos in the uterus fail to develop, another attempt can be made by unfreezing some of the frozen embryos and placing them in their mother's uterus. This technique means that the mother avoids a second abdominal operation.

Following IVF, about 10 per cent of women who are treated using this technique will give birth to a healthy baby.

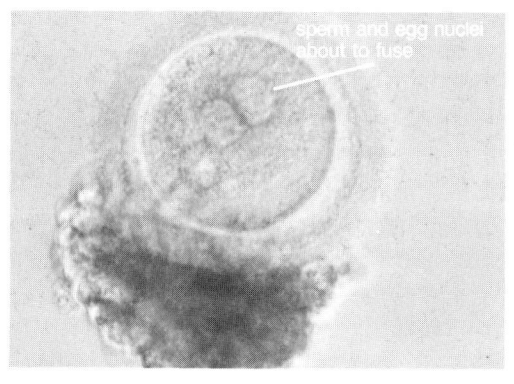

sperm and egg nuclei about to fuse

2

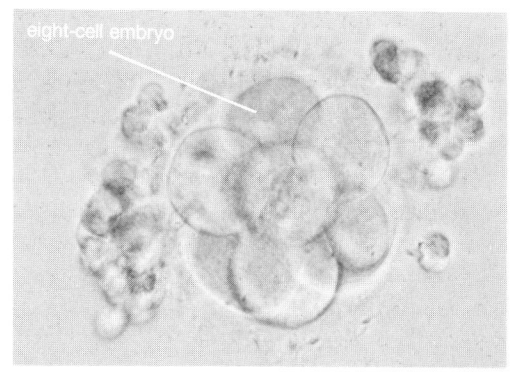

eight-cell embryo

5

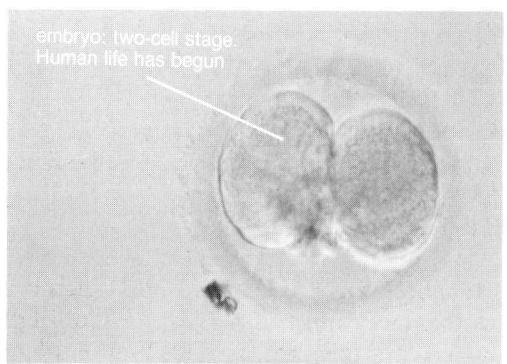

embryo: two-cell stage. Human life has begun

3

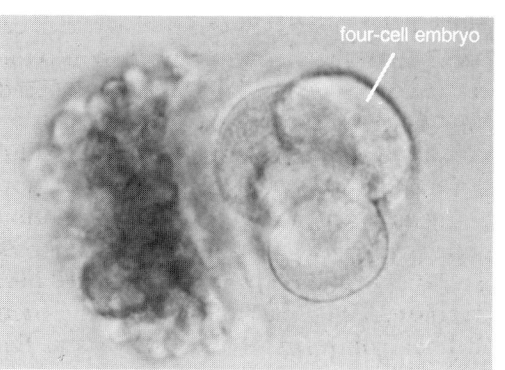

four-cell embryo

4

*Investigations*
- What are the procedures involved in adopting a baby in your State? Why do you think the number of babies available for adoption is decreasing?
- What is the procedure for donating and receiving sperm?
- Investigate the conditions necessary for a sperm and an egg to unite successfully outside the human body.
- Find out about the advantages and the disadvantages of in-vitro fertilization.

*Discussions*
- Discuss some of the implications for the child, the parents, and the donor of AID.
- Discuss your feelings about AID.
- Discuss your feelings about in-vitro fertilization.
- Looking at the sequence of photographs above, discuss when you think human life begins.

# 10

# SEXUALLY TRANSMITTED DISEASES

This group of infections, amongst which are the so-called venereal diseases, are called sexually transmitted diseases because they are spread almost exclusively by sexual contact. Usually they spread during vaginal sexual intercourse, but people can be infected after oral sex or after anal sex.

## The increase in sexually transmitted diseases and what to do about it

In the past twenty years the number of people infected by a sexually transmitted disease has increased dramatically. The greatest increase has been amongst young people, under the age of 25. As well, sexually transmitted diseases which previously were uncommon have become common, and diseases which were thought to be unimportant have become important. The diseases in order of frequency from the most common to the least common are: genital warts, non-gonococcal genital infection (including chlamydial infection), genital herpes, gonorrhoea, syphilis, and AIDS. As well, two common conditions which cause an annoying vaginal discharge in women—candidosis and trichomoniasis—often are transmitted sexually.

Why have the sexually transmitted diseases become so common?

The reasons for the rise in sexually transmitted diseases are complex. In part it is due to a more permissive attitude to sexual intercourse and to the increasing numbers of people who have sex with a casual partner. In part it is because the social and economic conditions in many countries have led to more people leaving home to work in other places or to go on holiday. In both these situations, people are more likely to make casual acquaintances to relieve loneliness or boredom. The chance acquaintance may lead to sexual intercourse with a partner who has a sexually transmitted disease.

A major problem in controlling the spread of two of the major diseases is that you may be infected and not know it. These two sexually transmitted diseases are non-gonococcal genital infection (NGGI) and gonorrhoea. The two sexually transmitted diseases affect the two sexes in different ways. NGGI usually causes a discharge from a man's penis; in a woman it usually does not cause a discharge from her urethra or her vagina. Instead the infection starts in her cervix and may cause no obvious symptoms. Gonorrhoea causes a discharge from a man's penis, and from the urethra of some women, but often the woman has no symptoms. This means that if a woman who is infected with either NGGI or gonorrhoea has sex with a new partner, he may be infected and then infect a new partner ... and so the diseases spread. It has been calculated that one-half of women who have been infected with

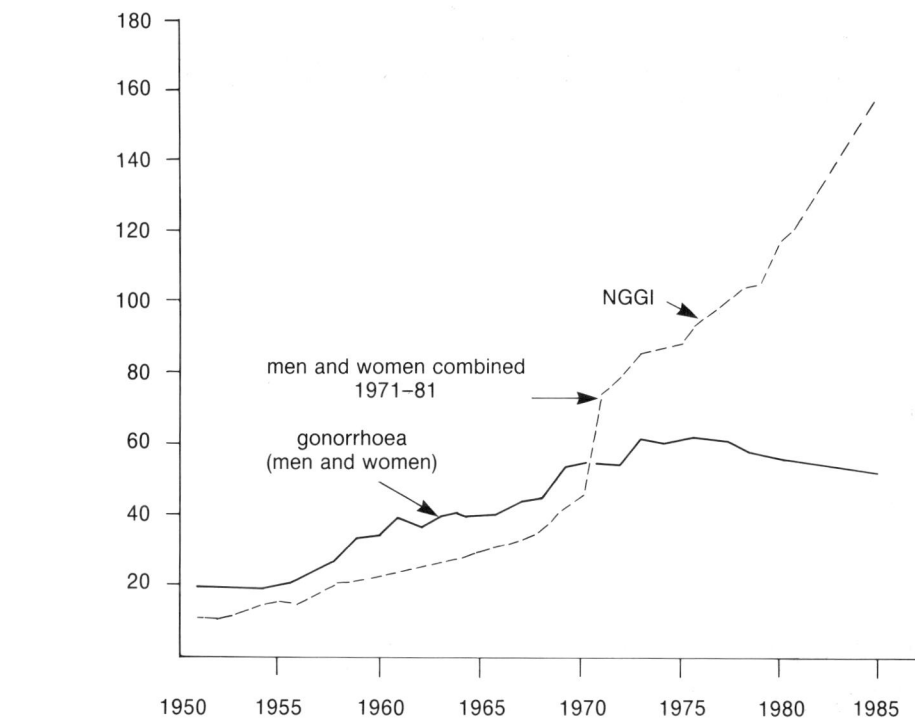

New cases of non-gonococcal genital infection (NGGI) reported in the United Kingdom since 1950

gonorrhoea and three-quarters of those infected with NGGI don't know that they have the sexually transmitted disease. It has also been calculated that, in men, one in ten who has gonorrhoea and one in five who has NGGI is unaware that he is infected.

The sexually transmitted diseases, including AIDS, could be eliminated if, all over all the world, no person had sex with anybody but his or her lifelong partner.

We have to be practical and realistic. We have to accept that casual sex will continue to occur. We have to be aware that an infected person who has sex with a new partner is likely to infect that person and that the spread of the sexually transmitted diseases will continue.

We can reduce the magnitude of the problem in two ways. First, we can change our attitude to sexually transmitted diseases. A person who has a 'sexual disease' is often ashamed because he or she feels guilty about it. Some of these people avoid getting treatment because of their shame and their fear of the doctor's reaction to them. If we treated sexually transmitted diseases like any other infectious diseases, the guilt and shame would go. This means, too, that people have to be less embarrassed about their sexuality.

A second way to reduce the spread of sexually transmitted diseases is for a woman to insist that the man wear a condom if she is unsure about his previous sexual behaviour. The reason for putting the responsibility on the woman is that she is affected more seriously by sexually transmitted diseases. NGGI and gonorrhoea may make a woman sterile, and the virus which causes genital warts may be a cause of cancer of the uterine cervix.

# Non-gonococcal genital infection

In about half of cases the infection is due to a small organism called chlamydia, and in the remainder it is due to a variety of organisms. Between 7 and 14 days (occasionally longer) after having sex, the man develops a creamy discharge from his urethra, and may have a burning sensation when he passes urine. Occasionally an infected woman has the same symptoms, but often, as I have mentioned, she has none.

If a person has symptoms and goes to the doctor, he or she takes a swab of the discharge, and it is sent to a laboratory. Unlike gonorrhoea, where characteristic small bean-shaped germs are found in pairs inside the pus cells, all that is found in NGGI are pus cells. If the doctor suspects chlamydia a test is now available to identify this organism.

In women, NGGI, especially if caused by chlamydia, may spread from the cervix to her uterus and then may infect her Fallopian tubes. The tubes may be so damaged that they become blocked, and this will prevent her becoming pregnant in the future. The more times a woman catches NGGI the greater the chance that this will occur. For this reason a woman who has sex with several partners would be wise to have medical checks at intervals.

A person who has NGGI diagnosed is treated by taking an antibiotic drug for about 7 days. During this period he or she should avoid alcohol and sex, because alcohol reduces the chance of cure and if sex takes place the partner may be infected and develop NGGI.

# Gonorrhoea

Gonorrhoea is one of the oldest diseases. It is mentioned in the Bible in Leviticus, the Third Book of Moses. It is spread almost exclusively by sexual contact either by vaginal intercourse, by oral sex, or by anal sex. It is *not* spread by 'picking it up from a lavatory seat'.

If you have sexual intercourse with an infected person, you have a sixty per cent chance of being infected by the small bean-like germs called **Neisseria gonorrhoea** which cause the disease. To remain alive the germ needs warmth, darkness, moisture, and an environment with just the right amount of oxygen. If it can't find these conditions it soon dies. It finds the right conditions in the human body, particularly in the cells which line the urethra (which is the tube connecting the bladder to the outside) and a woman's cervix. It can also thrive in the cells which line the tonsils and the rectum.

Between three and five days after being infected, a man notices a tingling discomfort in his urethra. Soon after this, a creamy, thick purulent (pus) discharge drips from his penis. He may also find it uncomfortable to pass urine, and when he does urinate, it burns.

A woman who has been infected with gonorrhoea may get the symptoms of burning and pain when she passes urine, or she may notice the appearance of a heavy, smelly, vaginal discharge.

The symptoms are due to the multiplication of the germ in the tissues of the urethra and a resulting inflammation.

If the infected person does not go for investigation and he or she has gonorrhoea, the infection spreads and the man or

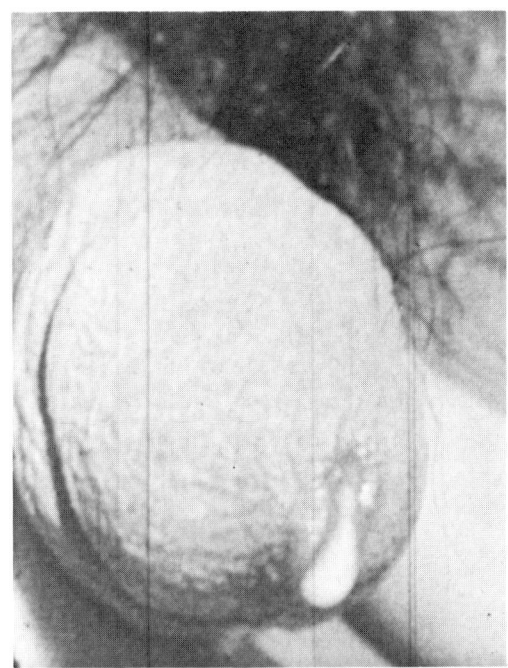

the woman may feel 'off colour'. Then the symptoms apparently settle down, and the person appears to be cured. Most people are cured, but without treatment early in the course of the disease there is a possibility that the germs may still be multiplying and causing damage. In a man, gonorrhoea may spread to his prostate gland or to his testicles, causing an acute inflammation and the chance of permanent damage. If this happens the man becomes sterile—he can never father children. If a woman fails to have treatment, the infection may spread downwards to infect a gland (Bartholin's gland) at the entrance to her vagina, causing a painful abscess; or it may spread upwards to her oviducts, damaging them, so that she can never bear a child.

These consequences can be avoided if people who think they may have gonorrhoea go for a check-up by a doctor.

The doctor takes a swab of the pus in the man's urethra, and from the urethra, the cervix and vagina of the woman. If the infected person says that he or she has had

This man has gonorrhoea. A bead of pus emerges from the 'eye' of the penis; when he passes urine it is painful. If the pus is examined under a microscope gonococci are found

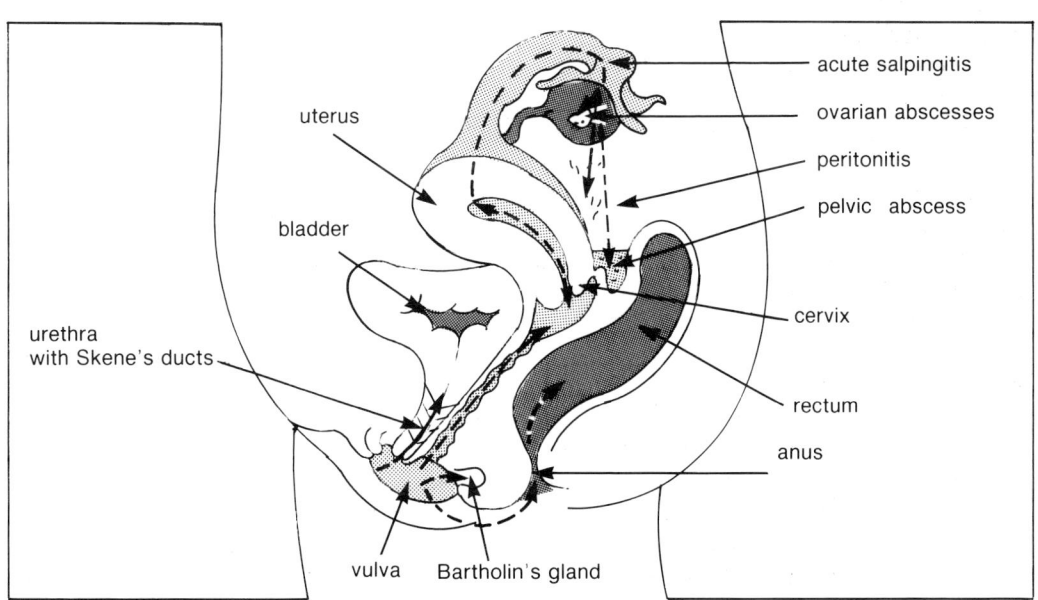

The spread of gonorrhoea in a woman

oral or anal sex, the doctor may also take swabs from the throat or anus.

The swabs are examined in the laboratory. If gonorrhoea is present, the bean-like germs are found lying in pairs within the pus cells.

Once the diagnosis has been made, the doctor will treat you with a penicillin injection or penicillin tablets, and ask you to take some other tablets as well. He will also ask you to try to get all your sexual contacts to come to be examined so that they can have the tests made and, if infected, be treated.

# Genital herpes

Most people know about and have had cold sores which form on the lips. They are due to a virus, called Herpes Simplex Virus Type 1. In recent years, a viral infection of the genital area of women and men has become increasingly common. In some cities it is now more common than gonorrhoea. The condition is genital herpes and it is usually due to a relative of the virus which causes cold sores. It is called Herpes Simplex Virus Type 2 (or HSV2), and is

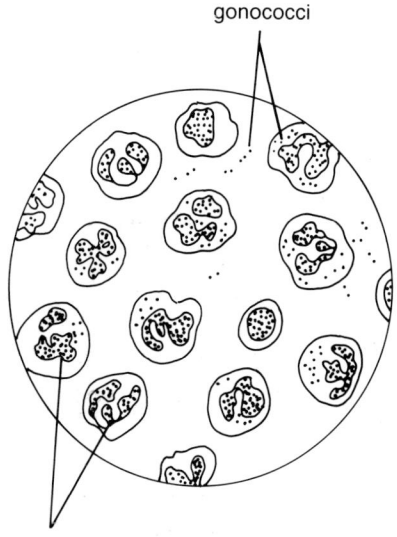

gonococci

nuclei of pus cells

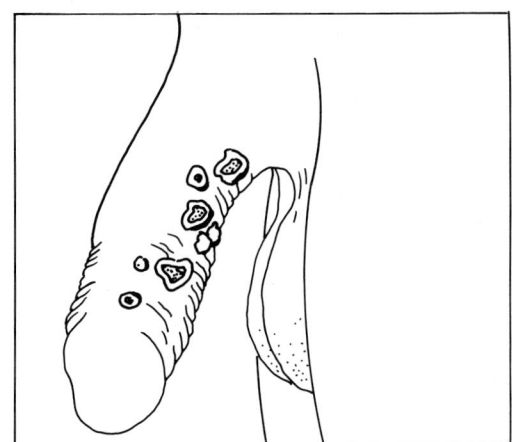

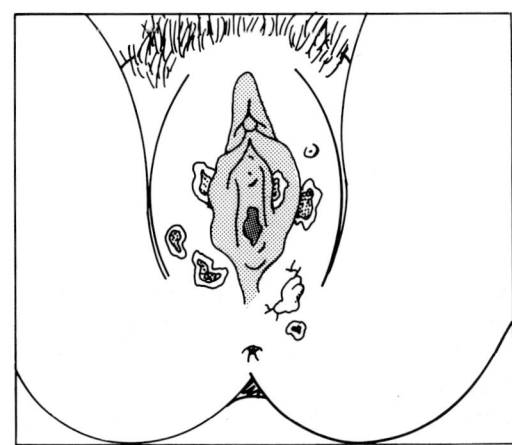

The painful, superficial ulcers of herpes on a man's penis and a woman's vulva

To be sure that you have been cured, you will have to go to the doctor for further check-ups each week for three weeks after you have had the penicillin treatment. It is worth it! After three weeks you know you are cured.

If the discharge persists during this time, you may have to take another type of antibiotic, as some varieties of the gonococcus are resistant to penicillin; or you may have also acquired non-gonococcal pelvic infection (NGGI) at the time you got gonorrhoea.

94

transmitted from person to person by sexual contact.

A few days after being infected by having sexual intercourse with a partner who has herpes blisters or ulcers on the genital area, you feel a localized burning on your genitals. In women, it is usually on the area round the entrance to the vagina. In men, the burning is felt on the shaft of the penis. The burning is followed by a collection of small blisters which burst to form shallow, very painful, ulcers. After a few days the ulcers form scabs, which eventually separate leaving a faint scar. The whole process lasts from seven to ten days. The herpes ulcers on a woman's vulva are very painful and often there is a lot of swelling as well, so that she may be unable to pass urine without great pain. In men the ulcers are also painful, but there is usually less swelling.

An unfortunate and often painful consequence of genital herpes is that about forty per cent of those infected have a second attack; and five per cent have recurrent attacks of herpes at longer or shorter intervals. The second and subsequent attacks are usually less painful, but even so can be very uncomfortable. Research is going ahead to produce drugs which will reduce the severity and duration of attacks of herpes. One, called acyclovir, is now available.

At present there is no cure for herpes. The ulcers heal in about seven days, but in some people recur after a long or short interval, when the whole painful process starts again.

No person infected with genital herpes should have sex until the ulcers have completely healed, or the person's partner will get the disease. A man should be especially careful, because if he infects a woman with HSV2 she may also get herpes on her cervix, and it is thought that this may be a factor in causing cancer of the cervix years later.

# Genital warts

Genital warts are becoming more common and are caused by a virus called the human papilloma virus. This virus is transmitted sexually. The warts may be quite small, especially on a man's penis, or larger, when they form cauliflower-like growths. In a woman they may form on her vulva, in her vagina, or on her cervix. It is believed that the virus may infect the cells of the cervix and lead years later to cancer. The changes to the cells can be detected by the Pap

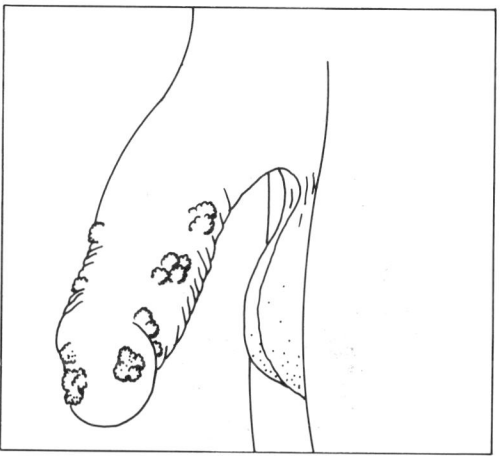
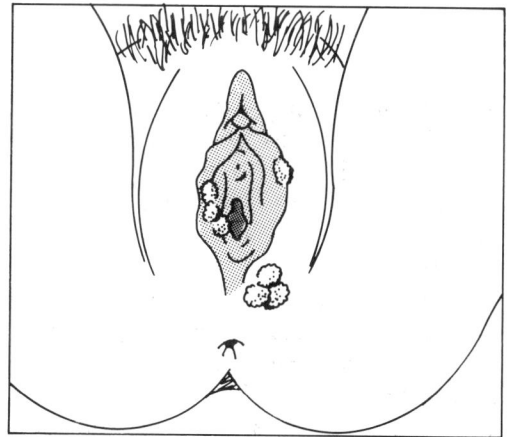

Genital warts on a man's penis and a woman's vulva

95

smear long before the cells become cancerous. It is important for a woman who doesn't know what her male partner's sexual behaviours have been to insist that he use a condom when they have sex.

Tiny warts on a man's penis can be detected by wrapping his penis in a vinegar-saturated cloth, when they will appear as white patches. These can be treated. Larger warts are obvious and can be cured by treating them with a drug which is painted onto each wart, or by burning them with a special instrument.

# Syphilis

Syphilis is the second least common of the major sexually transmitted diseases. It is a serious disease unless it is treated early and properly. Inadequately treated syphilis or untreated syphilis can cause damage to a person's heart, to the spinal cord, or to the brain. These rather horrible events only occur between ten and fifteen years after the first infection, and the man or woman with 'tertiary' syphilis either develops ulcerating tumours in the bones, a damaged heart, or goes slowly, horribly mad.

Syphilis is caused by a tiny pale corkscrew-like organism called **Treponema pallidum**. The germs enter the body through invisible abrasions in the skin or the soft delicate mucous membrane lining of the entrance to the vagina, the penis or other body openings (the mouth or the anus) which are used for sexual pleasuring. Once inside the body the germs multiply at a fantastic rate. They double their number every thirty hours, so if a person was infected with 1000 treponema, by the time symptoms appear the person has at least 10 000 million in the body.

The body tries to stem the invasion and mobilizes its defences. This takes time, and two to three weeks (sometimes up to twelve weeks) after a person was infected, a small

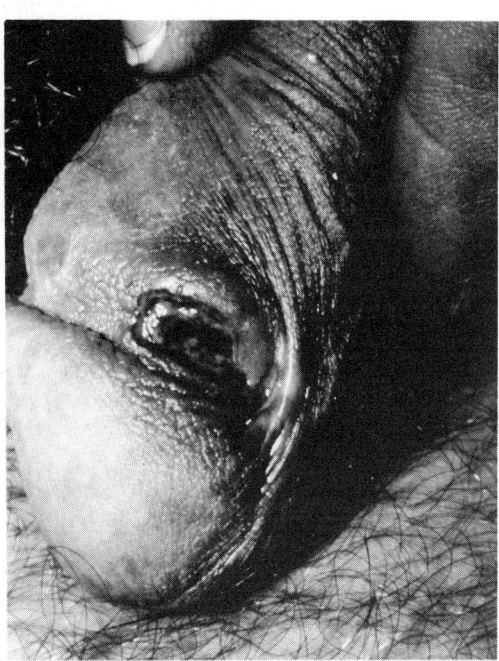

The first sign of syphilis on a man's penis—a chancre

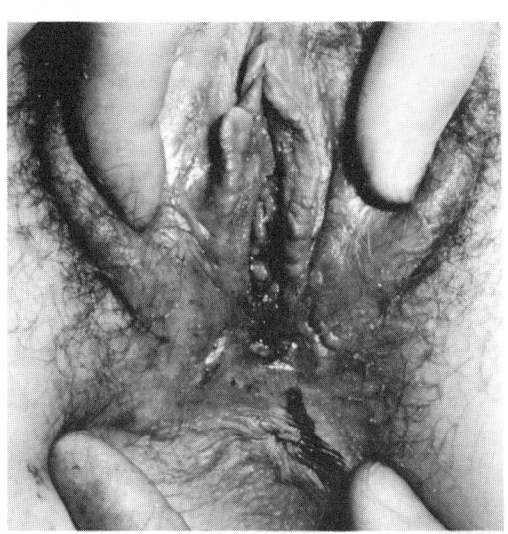

A chancre on a woman's vulva

red pimple develops, usually on a man's penis or on a woman's vulva. This becomes a hard, painless sore which oozes clear fluid. If the person has sexual intercourse with another person at this stage that person will be infected, as the fluid being discharged from the sore teems with treponema. The centre of the sore rots away, leaving a shallow ulcer with hard raised edges. This is the syphilitic chancre or 'hard sore'. At the same time the glands in the groins swell.

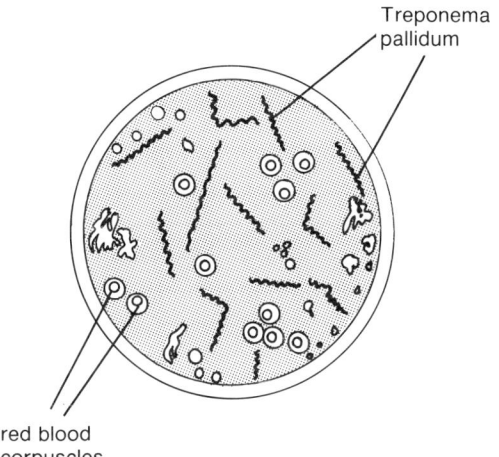

Treponema pallidum

red blood corpuscles

The cork-screw organisms which cause syphilis (*Treponema pallidum*) are seen in this smear taken from a chancre on a woman's labia

A smear taken from the chancre and examined under a microscope will show the corkscrew-like organisms which cause syphilis. Luckily, the organisms are very sensitive to penicillin, and provided a person cooperates fully with a doctor he or she will be cured. A daily injection of penicillin is given for between ten and twenty days. The person must continue to be seen by the doctor at intervals after the injections, so the doctor can be sure the person has been cured. This is checked by blood tests.

If no treatment is given at this, the first or primary, stage of syphilis, the sore slowly heals. Then, after a few weeks, the disease reappears, because the germs have been growing silently in the body, especially deep in the skin. First a widespread skin rash appears. It starts as pale pink spots which spread over the body and darken to a dusky red. The rash lasts for two or three weeks, the spots becoming pimples or pus spots. A few infected people develop shallow 'snail-track ulcers' in their mouth or on their vulva or in their anus. In women, flat-topped reddish warty growths may appear around the entrance to the vagina. By this time the body has made its defence against syphilis and the disease can be diagnosed by a blood test.

If the blood test is positive, penicillin will still cure the disease, but if you ignore the rash or the ulcers or the warts and don't get treatment, you have a fifty per cent chance of dying ten to twenty years later, in a rather horrible way, from tertiary syphilis.

# Sexually transmitted organisms which cause a vaginal discharge

Two organisms, one a small 'animal' and the other a fungus, are common causes of vaginal discharge and often are sexually transmitted. They are trichomonas vaginalis and candidosis.

## Trichomonas vaginalis

About ten per cent of women have this tiny little organism in their vagina. It causes an itchy vaginal discharge, and the woman's sexual partner may also be infected, but rarely has any symptoms. There is now a specific treatment which the woman and

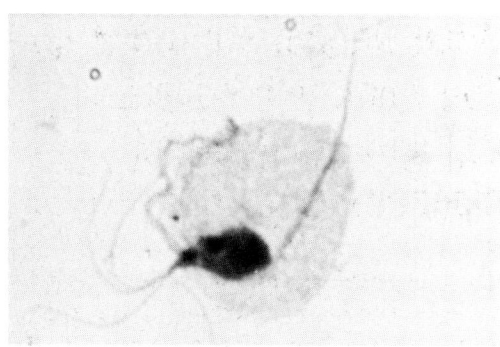

Trichomonads seen through a microscope

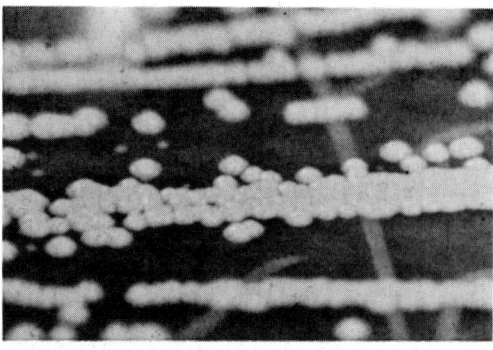

The filaments of *Candida albicans*,also called monilia or thrush, seen through a microscope

her sexual partner or partners should take. They take tablets of metronidazole every day for seven days or, if they prefer, a single large dose of the same tablets on one day.

## Candidosis

Vaginal candidosis or thrush is due to a fungus. It is much more common amongst sexually active women, and can be transmitted to their sexual partners. Candida causes a white or yellow vaginal discharge and, usually, a very itchy vulva. If a swab is taken and examined under a microscope, the threads of fungus can be seen. The treatment is to use vaginal tablets and ointment containing a fungus killer.

# AIDS

This new and frightening disease is caused by a virus, called the human immunodeficiency virus or HIV. HIV is usually transmitted during sexual intercourse, but may spread if drug addicts use the same needle for mainlining. A few cases have occurred following a blood transfusion.

In Central Africa, the AIDS virus has infected up to 30 per cent of the population, and is spread by having sex with prostitutes. In Western societies, most AIDS victims are homosexual men or drug addicts.

The word AIDS is derived from the **a**cquired **i**mmune **d**eficiency **s**yndrome. The term means that a person infected by HIV is more likely to develop severe, often fatal, infections which a non-infected person could shake off relatively easily.

Between 20 and 50 per cent of those infected with HIV will develop a chronic illness within five years. The illness makes the glands swell, produces fevers, and the person feels tired and often depressed.

This is called 'second stage AIDS' or the AIDS Related Complex. The person who has it either gets better or develops full-blown AIDS. If that happens he or she has an 80 per cent chance of dying from a severe pneumonia, some other severe infection, or a special kind of cancer, usually within a year.

● AIDS is not exclusively a homosexual disease.
● The virus is passed from person to person only in blood or in semen.
● You cannot get AIDS from casual contact.

● You cannot get AIDS from shaking hands, hugging or socially kissing an infected person.

● The virus is not transmitted if an infected person sneezes or coughs at you.

● You cannot get AIDS from sharing crockery, cutlery, towels or bed linen.

● You will not get AIDS if you swim in a place where an AIDS victim has swum.

● You cannot get AIDS from toilets, telephones or household furniture.

● You cannot get AIDS from non-sexual body contacts.

What of the future? Huge sums of money are being spent in many countries to find a vaccine which will prevent people being infected with the AIDS virus. None has yet been produced, but there is hope that one will be developed in the next five years.

A drug called Retrovir (or AZT) is available which makes a person who has full-blown AIDS much less ill and prolongs his or her life. Unfortunately the drug does not cure the disease.

At present the only way to control AIDS is for everyone to practise 'safer sex' and for drug addicts to stop sharing needles. Safer sex means having only one sexual partner, or using condoms if you don't know about your partner's previous sexual behaviour or have several sexual partners.

# What should you do if you think you have a sexually transmitted disease?

There is nothing to be ashamed about in having become infected with a sexually transmitted disease. What is antisocial, silly and dangerous to the community and to the person infected is to avoid going for help when the symptoms of the disease occur. If a person has no symptoms of any of these diseases but has multiple sexual partners, he or she should also get checked regularly.

*Discussions*

● What reasons can you think of for the spread of sexually transmitted diseases in most communities over the past few years?

● Discuss your ideas about ways of preventing the spread of sexually transmitted diseases.

● Discuss the myths about the spread of AIDS.

*Activities*

● Devise a community education campaign about sexually transmitted diseases.

## Sexually transmitted diseases

The major diseases in Western society:

● Non-gonococcal genital infection (NGGI), including non-gonococcal urethritis (NGU)

● Gonorrhoea

● Syphilis

● AIDS

The others:

● Herpes Simplex Virus Type 2

● Genital warts

● Trichomoniasis

● Candidosis

# 11
# ALTERNATIVE SEXUAL LIFESTYLES

Over 90 per cent of people form a relationship with a person of the complementary sex and most of these eventually marry. About 20 to 30 per cent of the marriages break down, and the couple separate, many obtaining a divorce. Marriage breakdown is more likely to occur if the couple have married when one or both were under the age of twenty, or when the marriage was 'forced' because of an unexpected pregnancy. After divorce, most of the divorced people either remarry or form a permanent or semi-permanent relationship with another partner.

About 10 per cent of people do not accept this conventional lifestyle, and form a relationship with a partner of the same sex (homosexuals); enjoy dressing in clothes usually worn by the other sex (transvestites); believe themselves to be of the other sex, imprisoned in the body of their own sex (transsexuals). There are also a number of people who have partners of each sex at different times during their lives (bisexuals).

## Homosexuality

A homosexual is a person who is 'turned on' sexually by a person of his or her own sex, in other words, has a sexual preference for someone of the same sex.

Apart from this erotic preference, almost all homosexuals are indistinguishable from heterosexual people. They are your neighbours. They may be doctors or dockers, packers or priests, lawyers or lumbermen, truck drivers or teachers, office-workers or artists.

Male homosexuals are no more likely to have a soft skin, a smooth face, feminine hands or gestures, than are heterosexual men. Female homosexuals, who are called lesbians, are no more likely to have a heavy build, a deeper voice, or other masculine characteristics than are heterosexual women. Apart from preferring a person of their own sex as a sexual partner, homosexual men and women have the same variety of interests and attitudes as heterosexual men and women.

There are a large number of homosexual men and women in the community. Reliable estimates suggest that one man in every twenty-five is homosexual by preference, and many more will have a homosexual relationship in certain situations, for example, when isolated in an all-male community. The number of female homosexuals (or lesbians) is not so certain, but at least one woman in every thirty is homosexual.

Ninety-five per cent of all homosexuals are indistinguishable from heterosexuals. Only five per cent, that is one homosexual in every twenty, fits the stereotyped image most people have of a homosexual. The stereotypical homosexual man wears flamboyant clothes, makes hand gestures, has limp wrists, speaks with a lisp, and minces as he walks. The stereotype lesbian is 'butch'; she wears man's clothes, is aggressive, heavy and loud. Those homosexuals who fit the stereotype do so because they feel comfortable in that role, or because they have been rejected or are insecure. At least the same proportion of heterosexual people behave in unconventional ways, because of feelings of rejection, wanting to attract attention, feeling insecure, or because they feel good when they behave in that way.

Homosexuality is not due to inherited influences. It is not due to a person having the wrong hormones. It is not an illness. Homosexuality usually becomes apparent in late childhood or early adolescence, when the person reaches the stage of making a choice of sexual partners; but a person may only be aware that he or she is homosexual much later on in life.

Homosexuality is not a perversion, nor is it a crime. Homosexuals are simply people who have an alternative sexual lifestyle.

Apart from their sexual relationships, homosexual men and women take part in similar activities, do similar jobs and enjoy similar entertainments to those of heterosexual men and women. Homosexual men and women have as many satisfying sexual relationships as heterosexual men and women. They may have sexual problems, but these are no more frequent than those of heterosexuals.

Relationships between homosexuals and children are usually gentle and full of concern; sexual assaults on the child are rare. In fact heterosexual assaults on children, ranging from rape, to incest, to bashing are far more common.

Many people fear homosexuality and despise homosexuals. In many countries the laws about homosexuality are repressive and homosexuals are harassed by the police. Homosexuals are mocked or derided in many films, plays and books. The hostility may make homosexuals feel

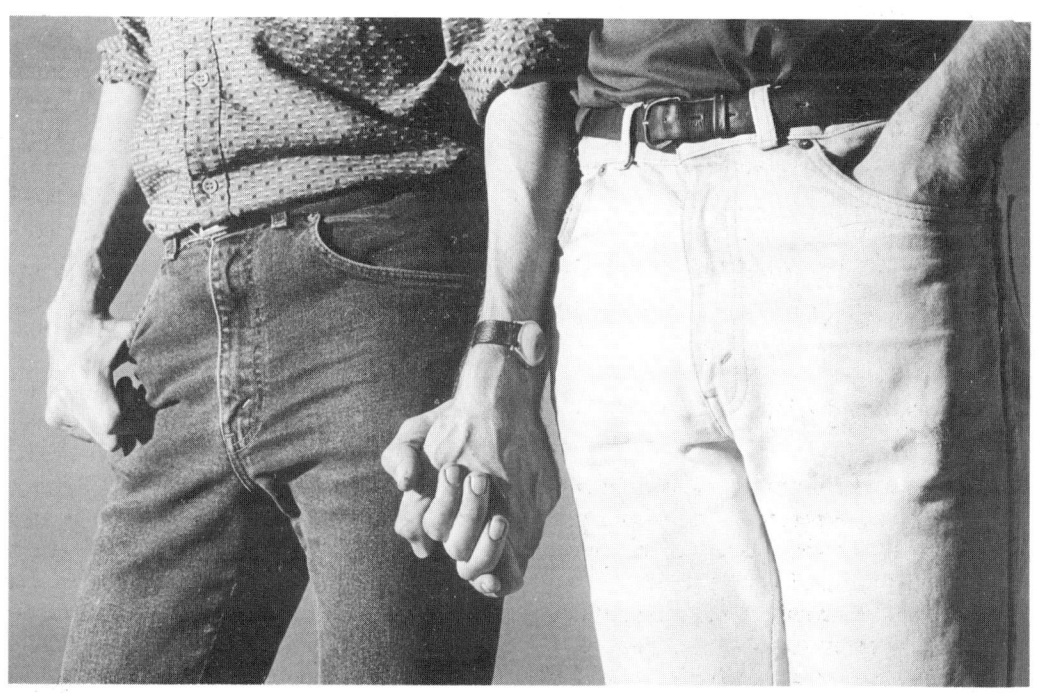

rejected, and fearful of being persecuted. Many react to this oppression by forming close-knit groups; others hide the fact that they are homosexual.

The condemnation of homosexuality by many people in society is damaging to the well-being and the health of at least one person in twenty in our nation.

### How do homosexuals make love?

Homosexual men and women enjoy body contact, they enjoy touching and pleasuring each other. As far as men are concerned it is probable that they are much more willing to pleasure their partner than are heterosexual men. Most homosexuals enjoy oral sex, as do many heterosexual men and women. Homosexual men also enjoy anal sex (as do some heterosexual men with their women partners). Contrary to popular belief, few homosexual men are exclusively the 'passive' partner, few are exclusively the 'active' partner during anal sex.

# Bisexuality (ambisexuality)

Bisexuals are people who, at some time or times in their lives, enjoy sexual experiences with people of their own sex; at other times they enjoy sexual experiences with people of the other sex.

In most cases a bisexual person has a warm supportive relationship with the partner of each sex, but sometimes a bisexual relationship is exploitive, as amongst some prison populations.

# Transsexuality

A transsexual is a person, usually a male, who appears in every physical sense to belong to one sex, but believes that he or she should belong to the other. The belief seems to begin about the time of puberty but many transsexuals have heterosexual relationships and experience sexual inter-

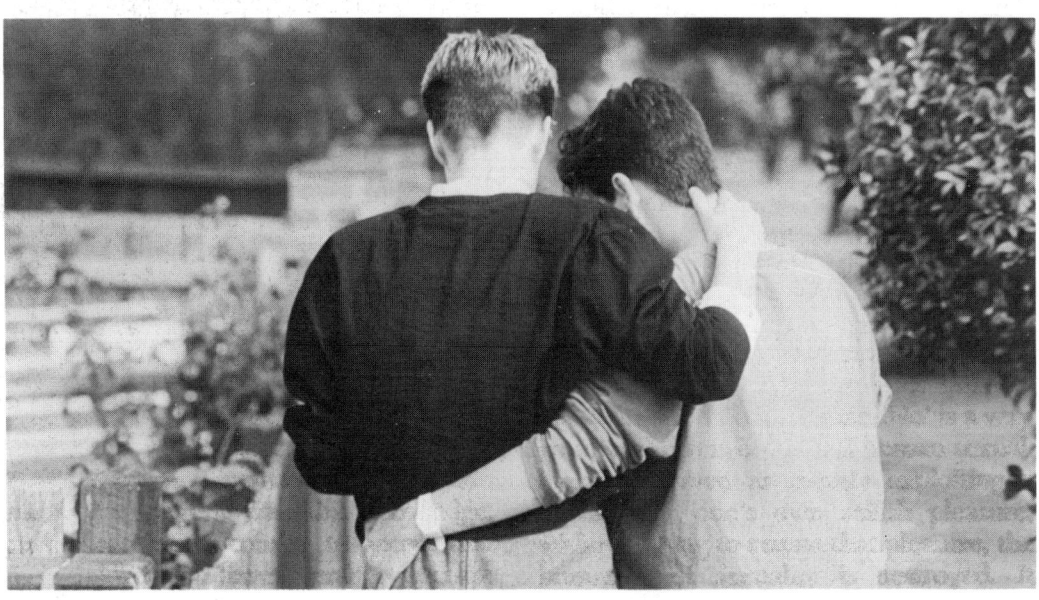

course. Some marry and have children before the strength of their belief that they are 'imprisoned in the body of a person of the other sex' drives them to seek help. Hormones are used to change the shape of the body to that of the desired sex; a man takes female sex hormones and grows breasts, a women takes male sex hormones and her breasts become flat. Some transsexual men also seek surgery to remove their penis and testicles and, later, to construct a vagina. The sex-change operations are painful and often unsuccessful, but receive a good deal of publicity. Surgery changes the physical appearance but the person still has to make the necessary psychological and emotional adjustments. Surgery is less important than other people's acceptance of the person's sex change.

A vivid description of transsexuals was written by Jan Morris in the book called **Conundrum**. Jan Morris, until her sex reassignment, was James Morris, a journalist who climbed Everest on the 1952 expedition and has travelled in many isolated and dangerous parts of the world. He was married and had children, with whom, as Jan, she now has a warm relationship.

# Transvestites

Transvestites, who are usually male, get pleasure from 'cross-dressing', that is from dressing in the clothes of the other sex, putting on make-up and then going out into public places and behaving the way the other sex conventionally behaves. Many children cross-dress, but only very few persist with the habit into adult life, becoming transvestites. Transvestites, when not engaged in cross-dressing, live normal heterosexual lives. Cross-dressing in childhood, or after, is not a sign of homosexuality. Not all transvestites cross-dress and go out. Many find sexual pleasure by cross-dressing at home, and then by masturbating.

# Fetishists

Fetishists are people (mainly men) who attach an important sexual significance to an object which is not necessarily sexual in itself. The fetish may be some part of the body such as the feet, or articles of clothing, such as shiny black leather boots, or frilly panties. Most people have preferences for parts of the body, or for certain clothes, colours, smells or tastes which stimulate them sexually. They are not fetishists. A fetishist is a person who is only aroused sexually by seeing, touching or fondling a particular part of the body or the particular garment for which he (or she) has a fetish.

*Investigations*
● What are the laws in your State governing alternative sexual expressions? Find out about their enforcement and compare them with the laws in other States and in other countries.
● Investigate public opinion in your community (school, family, neighbourhood etc.) about alternative forms of sexual expression.

*Discussions*
● Discuss your attitudes to homosexuality and consider how they have been formed.
● Discuss your attitudes to other forms of alternative sexual expression.

*Activities*
● Make a list of words synonymous with 'homosexual'. Comment about the usage of these words and how it relates to sex, culture, age, etc.

# 12
# RAPE

Rape is a particularly ugly sexual assault, usually on a woman or a child (although technically a man can be raped, for example, by other men in prison). A person is raped when she is forced to have sexual intercourse without her consent.

A rapist has contempt for women and treats them as objects, not as people. The man who rapes a woman may be a relative or someone she knows, or a stranger.

In recent years, as increasing numbers of women are prepared to face the indignity and, often, the humiliation of reporting that they have been raped, we have learned much more about rape.

● Rape doesn't necessarily mean that a stranger attacks a woman and drags her into a dark alley, the bush or a parked car. Nearly half of rapes are committed by a man known to the woman who rapes her in her own home.

● In many cases the woman lets the man into her home because she knows him; in others, the house is forcibly entered.

● Most rapes, and nearly all gang-rapes, are premeditated. The man, or gang of men, has planned to have sexual intercourse with the chosen woman, whether she consents or not.

● Most women who are raped are aged between twelve and forty-five, and most rapists are aged between sixteen and thirty-five.

At present, because of society's attitude to human sexuality, and because the woman is often exposed to humiliation by the police when she reports the case, and later by the defence lawyer in court, most cases of rape are not reported. All too often when a woman reports that she has been raped her story is not believed, and she is thought to have encouraged the man or to have 'loose morals'.

A common defence of a rapist is that the woman 'incited' him to rape her because she was wearing 'provocative' clothes, or because she behaved in a 'seductive' way or because she made 'suggestive' remarks. The implication is that the woman was responsible by her behaviour for unleashing an uncontrollable sexual urge in the man.

Even if the statements made by rapists were true, and all the evidence is that they are not, a man who cannot control himself sexually, when he finds that the woman does not want sexual intercourse, is sick.

## Who are rapists?

Although rapists are sick people they are usually not mentally disturbed.

Their sickness is caused, in part, by the way society conditions males to behave. In our society, men are taught to be aggressive and tough; they are taught to 'hunt' women as they might hunt animals. Men are taught that they have a higher, more urgent, sex drive than women, and that once aroused the drive is so strong that it is a struggle to control the urge for sex. Men are taught that women are and should be submissive and passive in their relations with men. They are dependent on men. They have a lower sexual drive than men, they need sex less often and with less urgency, but really they incite men to have sex.

These myths about male and female sexuality, which are widely believed, are untrue. The difference in the sexual behaviour of men and women is due not to biological differences but to the way boys and girls are reared and to what they learn about sexuality.

Society has conditioned men to believe that they are sexual predators, that women really want to have sex but are too shy to ask, and that men should subdue women sexually. The rapist sees himself as the wolf or tiger, and he sees the woman as the prey, the chick or the bird.

Most rapists are insecure in their relations with other people. They feel a need to prove their masculinity, their machismo. They get excitement from causing fear and pain. They get excitement from feeling powerful, from subjugating and humiliating the woman. One rapist recently said, 'I despise women who give in to me and I hate them if they don't.'

# What are the effects of being raped?

Every woman who has been raped is distressed; she feels 'used'. The physical effects may be painful and the emotional damage even more so. Luckily, such is the human capacity for mental resilience, the trauma passes away fairly quickly; but fears can remain, and may damage the woman's sexuality for years. The physical damage may include bruises and tears of the woman's vagina; worse, she may be infected by a sexually transmitted disease, or may be made pregnant.

Recovery from the effect of being raped is quicker and easier if, as soon as possible after being raped, the woman can talk to a sympathetic, supportive person, who believes her story and who treats her as a human being.

# What should you do if you are raped?

If you are raped you should tell a responsible person—your parents, or a close friend—as soon as possible after the rape, so that they can support you and be a witness to your emotional state.

In some countries rape crisis centres have been started. These are run by trained, concerned, sympathetic people and provide additional support, both mental and physical, to a woman who has been raped.

After being able to share your distress you may choose to report the rape to the police. If you do, you can lessen the humiliation and the unpleasantness of talking to strangers by doing certain things before you report that you have been raped.

First, try to remember exactly what took place, and in what order. When you tell the police be as matter-of-fact as you can.

Second, do not shower, wash your vulva, or change your appearance or your clothes, until you have been examined by a doctor. The doctor has to look for evidence of assault, or injury to your body, for bruises, and scratches, and he or she will have to look at your genital organs to see if there is any injury and to find if there are any sperms. The police may want to keep your clothes as evidence, so take clean clothes with you.

Third, don't drink any alcohol. The police may smell the alcohol and it may lead to the claim that you were drunk when the rape took place.

Fourth, the police usually work rather slowly. They may disbelieve your story and give you a hard time trying to find out if the rape really happened. But it is their job to find out and this is their way of finding out. So be prepared for a long stay at the police station. Rape crisis centres will help to improve matters considerably.

Fifth, if the case comes to trial, the defence lawyer may try to destroy your character by making out that you are promiscuous or a liar, so that he can prove that you incited his client to have sex with you. It is your word against the defendant's because few rapes are witnessed—except for gang-rapes, when all the men involved deny that the rape occurred.

*Investigations*
● Find out all you can about rape crisis centres and the facilities they are offering.

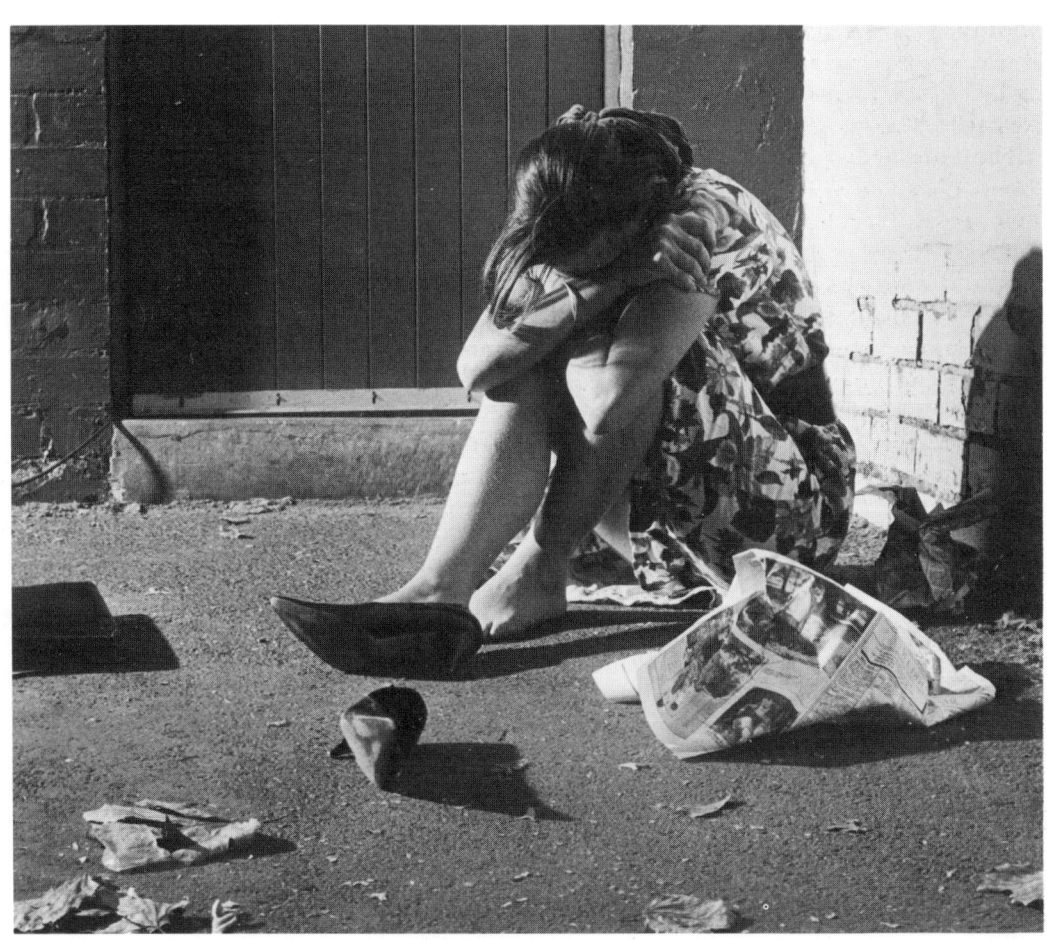

# 13
# SEXUAL PROBLEMS AND THEIR SOLUTION

An important finding of Michael Schofield's 1966 survey of adolescent sexual behaviour in Britain was that more than half of sexually active teenagers were anxious about, or dissatisfied with, their sexuality.

Seven years later he resurveyed many of the teenagers, who were now aged twenty-five. Four people out of every ten with whom he talked felt that their knowledge of sex was inadequate. He observed, 'It is the lack, not the surfeit of knowledge that is the cause of distress'.

The main concerns the young adults had about their sexuality were: anxiety about their sexual performance, guilt about having sex at all, anxiety about masturbation, and boredom with sex.

Other investigations have shown that a considerable number of young men are worried that their penis is smaller than it should be, or that their acne is due to masturbation, dirtiness or 'bad blood'. A number of young women are worried about the size of their breasts (aren't they too small or too big?) or that their vagina is too small so that when they have sexual intercourse it will be painful.

These anxieties can be eliminated by knowing more about sexuality.

## Sexual performance problems

When a person is not performing sexually as well as he or she would wish, the person is said to have a sexual dysfunction.

Most sexual problems occur amongst adults rather than teenagers, but some teenagers are worried about their sexual performance.

Three sexual dysfunctions occur amongst men and women and may be more common than many people believe.

## Sexual problems amongst men

The most common sexual problem amongst men is prematue ejaculation. The man is aroused so much that he ejaculates either before or very soon after starting sexual intercourse. In this way he reduces his own sexual pleasure and may prevent his partner from fully enjoying sex.

The second, and least common problem, is the reverse. The man enjoys making love, he enjoys sexual intercourse, but no matter how hard or long he tries, he just cannot reach orgasm.

The third problem is the most destructive to a man's masculinity. This is when he finds he can no longer get or sustain an erection. He believes that he is a failure as a man and as a lover because instead of a hard, erect penis, all he has is a limp, floppy organ. He has become impotent.

Most men find that from time to time they cannot get an erection when they want to, but an impotent man finds that he cannot ever get an erection. And it worries him a great deal.

Impotence may be due to disease (especially diabetes) or to drugs given for treatment of illness. It may be due to drinking too much alcohol (it is called 'brewer's droop'), but in many cases it is due to anxiety or to depression.

# Women's sexual problems

The first of the sexual problems that affects women is not being aroused sexually by their partner. A woman may dislike the idea of having to have sexual intercourse, with the result that her vagina does not lubricate.

The second problem is that the woman wants to have sexual intercourse but is unable to, because every time the man tries to put his penis in her vagina it hurts her. What actually happens is that fear or anxiety causes her to tighten the muscles around her vaginal entrance so much that the man hurts her trying to have sex. This is called vaginismus.

The third problem is that although the woman wants sex, enjoying the feel of her partner's body against her, and of his penis within her vagina, she fails to have an orgasm whilst he is thrusting in her vagina. Many people now feel that this is a problem because of the widespread false belief that for sex to be normal a woman must have an orgasm during sexual intercourse. Only half of women do, but nearly every woman can have an orgasm if the man caresses her clitoris with his finger, or with his tongue in oral sex, or if she masturbates.

# The solutions

Most sexual problems can be solved, and many will not arise, if people can learn to talk to each other about their sexuality. The earlier in a relationship that this starts, the greater is the chance that problems will be prevented.

Teenagers can start this communication by finding out their partners' needs, and by respecting their partners' wishes. They can learn to pleasure each other and, when they are relaxed, to talk specifically about their desires, their feelings and their expectations. Many young women feel embarrassed to ask their partner to give them sexual enjoyment in a particular way. Many young men believe that their sexual needs are so urgent that what the woman feels is unimportant. Communication between the couple will change these feelings and make the relationship much deeper, fuller and more pleasurable.

# Sex and the spinal cord injured

One of the most common serious injuries which happens to young people is an injury to the spinal cord following an automobile accident or an accident in sport.

Imagine that you have had a spinal injury. Suddenly you have become paralysed and can feel nothing from the waist down. You have no control over your bladder or your bowels. Your bladder empties through a tube to a plastic bag strapped to your leg. Regularly, without knowing it, you empty your bowels. You have no feeling in your genitals or your legs. Your lower body and legs go into spasms, often several times a day.

When you leave hospital, you will only be able to move about in a wheelchair. To talk to people you have to tilt your head back and look up.

The muscles of your legs and buttocks waste away and you may become self-conscious about your body.

As a healthy young person, you enjoyed masturbating or making love; suddenly

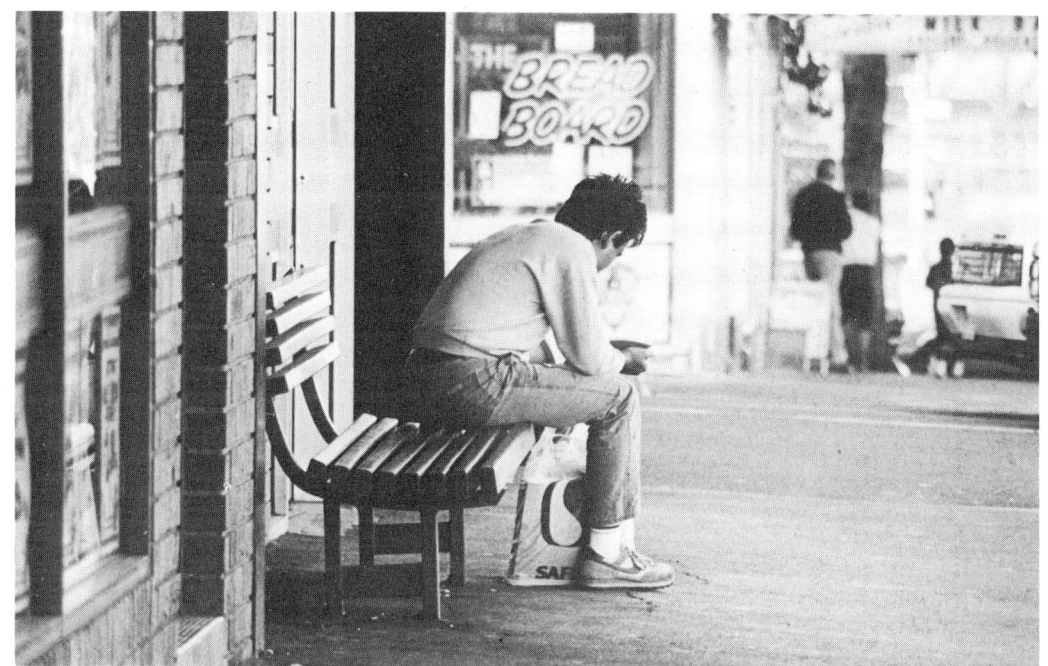

you find that you have no sensations from your genitals and become worried about whether you can ever enjoy your sexuality, or whether you are to be condemned to a life of celibacy.

You can enjoy your sexuality, provided that you have a partner who loves you, and have proper counselling. Most paraplegic men can get erections and, although they can feel nothing, get pleasure from their partner's pleasure during sexual intercourse. They also obtain pleasure from touching and cuddling their partner. Most paraplegic women repond to the partner's stimulation of their genitals although they feel nothing. The woman gets pleasure from seeing her partner's pleasure during sexual intercourse, or if she has oral sex with him. She gets pleasure from cuddling, from breast stimulation and from being in a warm relationship. She can also become pregnant and give birth to a healthy baby.

A paraplegic man usually cannot ejaculate so that the likelihood of him fathering a baby is small, although new techniques of obtaining sperm from him may change this.

Given proper help there is no reason today why a spinally injured man or woman should not continue to enjoy an active sex life.

## Sex and the disabled

People who have no physical or mental disabilities believe that those people who are mentally retarded, or are paralysed, or physically damaged, neither want nor need sex. They are treated as non-persons because of their disability. The truth is that disabled people can enjoy sex, and should be given the opportunity to have sex if they want it. Through their sexuality they can relate to another person and can enjoy the closeness and intimacy of being with that person. That is what human sexuality is. It is unity and harmony with another person so that both benefit. It is intimate communication with another person. It is closeness and mutual pleasuring of body and mind.

# Sex and age

Many young people believe that as a person grows older the desire and need for sex is reduced. This is untrue; older people continue to enjoy their sexuality. As a man grows older it takes him longer to get an erection; he takes longer to reach orgasm; and he needs a longer interval between the times he can ejaculate. A woman's sexual drive does not change so much as she grows older; in fact it often increases.

Most people enjoy sex as they grow older as much, or more, than they did when they were young, but there is a difference between men and women. Women go on enjoying sex until they are very old. Older men, particularly over the age of seventy, often find it more difficult to get an erection and have sexual intercourse. This does not prevent them enjoying touching, caressing and being close to their partner, in a warm relationship. There are wide individual variations. Some men of eighty enjoy sexual intercourse regularly; some men of sixty are less able to become sexually aroused, in spite of being stimulated.

It is known that the more a man or a woman enjoyed their sexuality and the more that they were able to relate sexually when they were young, the greater is the chance that they will enjoy sex into old age.

*Investigations*
● Investigate the incidence of physical disability as a result of road accidents in the fifteen to twenty-five age group.

*Discussions*
● Discuss the difficulties encountered by a disabled person in the expression of his or her sexuality. How do you think such a person can be helped by the community to overcome these difficulties?

*Activities*
● Write a description of yourself as you would like to be when you are an old person.

## Anxieties about sex by sexually active young adults

|  | Men | Women |
|---|---|---|
| ● Worry about sexual performance | 21% | 13% |
| ● Boredom in sex | 7% | 16% |
| ● Guilt about having sex | 21% | 15% |
| ● Anxiety about masturbation | 12% | 2% |

Schofield, M. *The Sexual Behaviour of Young Adults*, Allen Lane, London, 1973.

# GLOSSARY AND EVERYDAY WORDS

| | |
|---|---|
| Anal intercourse | buggery, sodomy. |
| Anus | the outlet of the bowel, also known as: arse, arse-hole, bum, back passage. |
| Breasts | boobs, knockers, tits, norgs. |
| Cervix | the 'neck' or lowest part of the uterus, which projects into the vagina. |
| Clitoris | the small sensitive organ which is found in the front part of a woman's vulva; it equates to the penis, and its stimulation leads to orgasm; also called: clit, button or bud. |
| Contraceptives: | |
|   Condom | rubber, french letter, franger, sheath. |
|   Diaphragm | Dutch cap. |
| Cunnilingus | the act of licking or sucking the clitoris; also called: cunt-sucking, eating, going down on, head job. |
| Ejaculation | the discharge of semen from the penis after sexual stimulation; also called: coming, dropping a load, jacking off, shooting a wad, etc., etc. |
| Erection | the physiological change which occurs to the penis from sexual stimulation; also called: a hard on, a horn, a stand. |
| Fellatio | the act of sucking a penis; also called: cock-sucking, a blow job, a head job. |
| Gender role | everything a person says or does which indicates to other people that the person is a male or female, or ambivalent; also called sex role, but as the term sex is used in so many different ways, gender role is less confusing. |
| Gender identity | the firm conviction based on self-awareness and behaviour that a person is male, female or ambivalent; it is the private expression of the gender role. |

111

| | |
|---|---|
| Gonorrhoea | a sexually transmitted disease;<br>also: clap, dose. |
| Heterosexual | a person whose erotic (sexual) preference is for a member of the other sex. |
| Homosexual | a person who has an erotic preference for someone of his or her own sex. |
| Female homosexual | a dyke, a gay, a femme, or a lesbian. |
| Male homosexual | fairy, faggot, fag, nancy, poofter, queen, queer, gay. |
| Impotent | to be unable to obtain or maintain an erection;<br>also called: with brewer's droop, droopy, limp. |
| Masturbate | to stimulate one's own penis or clitoris;<br>also called: to beat off, hand-job, jerk-off, pull the pudding, pull Percy, wank. |
| Menstruation | curse, dog days, rags on, period. |
| Orgasm | the climax of sexual arousal;<br>a pervasive, warm, wonderful sensation which spreads from the pelvis to fill the whole body; during orgasm, every other sensation is obliterated, it overwhelms everything;<br>also called: a climax, a crisis, or 'coming'. |
| Oviducts | the narrow tubes which stretch from the uterus towards the ovaries;<br>also called: 'the Fallopian tubes'. |
| Penis | the male external sexual organ;<br>also called: cock, donger, John Thomas, nob, pecker, prick, one-eyed trouser-snake, wanger, dick, etc., etc. |
| Pregnant | in the club, expecting, in the family way, (have a) bun in the oven, up the spout. |
| Promiscuous (person) | only seems to apply to women;<br>also called: anybody's, dead cert, easy lay, easy make, scrubber, swinger, slut, etc., etc. |
| Pubic hair | beaver, bush, fuzz, mult, thatch. |
| Rectum | the back passage;<br>also called: bum gut. |
| Semen | the material which is ejaculated from a man's penis;<br>also called: cum (come), load, juice, jism, spunk, wad. |

| | |
|---|---|
| Scrotum | the sack of skin in which a man's testicles are found—his ball-bag. |
| Sexual intercourse (to have) | to bang, to dip the wick, to fuck, to hump, to knock, to lay, to poke, to roger, to shag, to shaft, to screw, to have a naughty, to have some nooky. |
| Syphilis | a sexually transmitted disease; also called: the pox. |
| Testicles (Testes) | the two organs in which spermatozoa and the male hormone testosterone are made; also called: cobblers, balls, bollocks, goolies, marbles, nuts. |
| Virgin (to have intercourse with a) | a woman who has never had sexual intercourse; also called: a cherry, to take the cherry. |
| Vulva | a woman's external sexual organs; also called: bearded clam, crack, cunt, hole, nook (nooky), poon tang, pussy. |

# FURTHER READING

ABRAHAM, Suzanne and LLEWELLYN-JONES, Derek. *Eating Disorders—The Facts.* 2nd edn. Oxford University Press, Oxford, 1987.

ALTMANN, Denis. *Homosexual.* Penguin, Ringwood, 1971.

BELLIVEAU, Fred and RICHTER, Lin. *Understanding Sexual Inadequacy.* Bantam, New York, 1970.

BOSTON WOMEN'S HEALTH BOOK COLLECTIVE. *The New Our Bodies, Ourselves.* Penguin, Harmondsworth, 1984.

LLEWELLYN-JONES, Derek. *Everywoman.* 4th edn. Faber, London, 1986.

LLEWELLYN-JONES, Derek. *Everyman.* 2nd edn. Oxford University Press, Oxford, 1987.

LLEWELLYN-JONES, Derek. *Herpes, AIDS and Other Sexually Transmitted Diseases.* Faber, London, 1985.

LLEWELLYN-JONES, Derek and ABRAHAM, Suzanne. *Everygirl.* Oxford University Press, Melbourne, 1986.

MAYLE, Peter. *What's Happening to Me?* Sun Books, Melbourne, 1978.

NILSSON, Lennart. *A Child is Born.* Faber, London, 1974.

SCHOFIELD, Michael. *The Sexual Behaviour of Young People.* Penguin, Harmondsworth, 1967.

SCHOFIELD, Michael. *The Sexual Behaviour of Young Adults.* Allen Lane, London, 1973.

TUOHY, Felicity and MURPHY, Michael. *Down under the Plum Trees.* Alister Taylor Ltd., New Zealand, 1976.

TRIPP, C. A. *The Homosexual Matrix.* Signet, New York, 1975.

WEST, Donald. *Homosexuality.* Penguin, Harmondsworth, 1971.

# ACKNOWLEDGEMENTS

The author wishes to acknowledge the assistance of Anne Mulholland and Lawrence St. Leger of the Social Biology Resources Centre, Carlton, Vic. in evaluating the manuscript from an educational perspective and for providing the end-of-chapter activities.

The following extracts were reproduced with the publishers' permission: Table of anxieties about sex by sexually active young adults, from Michael Schofield: *The Sexual Behaviour of Young Adults* (Allen Lane, 1973) pp. 175–76. © Michael Schofield, 1973. Reprinted by permission of Penguin Books Ltd.

Table of findings about childhood sexuality, from A. Gesell and P. Ilg: *The Child from Five to Ten* (Harper & Row, Publishers, Inc., 1977), abridged and adapted from pp. 311–314 in *The Child from Five to Ten*, revised edition by Arnold Gesell, Frances L. Ilg and Louise Bates Ames. Copyright 1946 by Arnold Gesell and Frances L. Ilg; renewed 1974 by Gerhard A. Gesell, Katherine Gesell Walden and Frances L. Ilg. Copyright © 1977 by Louise Bates Ames, Frances L. Ilg and Glenna E. Bullis. Reprinted by permission of Harper & Row, Publishers, Inc.

The author and publisher also wish to thank the following: John Brennan for the photographs on pages 2, 4, 20, 27, 29, 31, 36, 37, 38, 42, 51, 56, 57, 58, 59, 61, 78, 83, 101, 102, 106 and 109; Rennie Ellis for the photographs on page 5; Gary Tregaskis for the photograph on page 6; The Family Planning Association, Queensland, for the photograph on page 54; The Women's Hospital, Crown Street, Sydney, for the photographs on page 74 and 77; Helen Grace for the photographs on page 81; Prue Carr (photographer) and Susan and Adam Crocket (models) for the photograph on page 84; Beecham Research Laboratories for the photographs on pages 93 and 98; Monash Medical Centre for the photographs on page 96; and Professor D. Saunders and the IVF team of the Royal North Shore Hospital, Sydney, for the photographs on pages 88 and 89.

# INDEX